W9-BND-089

DATE DUE

The Quantum Leader
Applications for the New World of Work

Kathy Malloch, PhD, MBA, RN, FAAN
President
Kathy Malloch Consulting Services
Glendale, Arizona

Faculty Associate, College of Nursing
Arizona State University
Tempe, Arizona

Vice President
Arizona State Board of Nursing

Evidence Based Researcher
Banner Estrella Medical Center
Phoenix, Arizona

Tim Porter-O'Grady, EdD, PhD, FAAN
Senior Partner
Tim Porter-O'Grady Associates, Inc.
Atlanta, Georgia

Associate Professor
Emory University
Atlanta, Georgia

JONES AND BARTLETT PUBLISHERS
Sudbury, Massachusetts
BOSTON   TORONTO   LONDON   SINGAPORE

World Headquarters
Jones and Bartlett Publishers
40 Tall Pine Drive
Sudbury, MA 01776
978-443-5000
info@jbpub.com
www.jbpub.com

Jones and Bartlett Publishers Canada
6339 Ormindale Way
Mississauga, ON L5V 1J2
CANADA

Jones and Bartlett Publishers
International
Barb House, Barb Mews
London W6 7PA
UK

ISBN-13: 978-0-7637-2912-7
ISBN-10: 0-7637-2912-4

Library of Congress Cataloging-in-Publication Data

Malloch, Kathy.
  The quantum leader : applications for the new world of work / Kathy Malloch, Tim Porter-O'Grady.
      p. ; cm.
  Includes bibliographical references and index.
  ISBN 0-7637-2912-4 (pbk. : alk. paper)
  1. Leadership. 2. Nursing services—Administration. 3. Psychology, Industrial.
  [DNLM: 1. Leadership. 2. Nursing, Supervisory. 3. Psychology, Industrial. WY 105 M255q 2005] I. Porter-O'Grady, Timothy.
II. Title.
HD57.7.M348 2005
658.4'092—dc22

                                                                                        2004021984

6048

Production Credits
Acquistions Editor: Kevin Sullivan
Production Director: Amy Rose
Associate Production Editor: Renée Sekerak
Associate Editor: Amy Sibley
Senior Marketing Manager: Ed McKenna
Associate Marketing Manager: Emily Ekle
Manufacturing and Inventory Coordinator: Amy Bacus
Composition: Auburn Associates, Inc.
Cover Design: Kristin E. Ohlin
Printing and Binding: Courier Stoughton
Cover printing: Courier Stoughton

Printed in the United States of America
10 09 08 07 06   10 9 8 7 6 5 4 3 2

Contents

Chapter 8   The Leader as Mentor and Coach

Chapter 9   Leading with Courage

Chapter 10 Leadership and Care of the Self

Foreword

Since the work of leadership is ever changing and yet still the same in many ways, *The Quantum Leader* is written for both current and aspiring leaders as a means to gain an appreciation of the complexities faced today. New strategies, new behaviors, and of course, new vulnerabilities are required to practice in the evolving world of technology, while health-care leaders are challenged to consistently sustain system infrastructures that support the essential caring and therapeutic behaviors of the healer.

In writing this book, the interconnectedness of leadership behaviors was consistently challenging and revealing. Writing about behaviors that were undeniably connected and intertwined challenged us as we attempted to clarify concepts without creating artificial boundaries between them. Necessarily, a vulnerable leader must be courageous, a peacemaker who is continually challenged to minimize toxic behaviors. Coaching in the new age requires full engagement in order to achieve therapeutic and value-based services.

The Quantum Leader is written from the perspective of the health-care leader and healer but has applications to leadership in any discipline that is accountable for the work of facilitation of others, coaching for achievement, elimination of toxic behaviors, and leading into the future. We invite leaders in all organizations to share in our work and as always to share ideas and suggestions to improve the work of the quantum leader.

Kathy Malloch
Tim Porter-O'Grady

Acknowledgments

Writing this book has added much to my life. I have continued to expand my thinking about leadership and to appreciate the importance of competent and authentic leaders. My journey in health care has been blessed with a most supportive family and very special friendships of the best and brightest professionals. Much recognition goes to Bryan E. Malloch, D.O., my best friend, my confidant and my husband. He has never wavered in his support and recognition of my endeavors—even those classified as *wild hairs*! Having Tim Porter-O'Grady as a mentor, colleague and friend is a gift that I cherish every day, and I hope to continually learn from his wisdom, love of excellence, and willingness to listen to new ideas. Finally, I would like to acknowledge my dad, Joe Fox, who passed away March 5, 2004, after four years in a nursing home. He instilled a strong work ethic in me, a desire for excellence, and continuous motivation to develop better personal relationship skills—skills that he himself always struggled to achieve. I will continue to be influenced by his positive qualities, challenged by his shortcomings and always strive to be the best that I can be. Thank you, Dad—I love you for who you were.

Kathy Malloch

My thanks and appreciation to Mark Ponder who continues to exemplify the best in caring and nursing, demonstrating the reality that gender has nothing to do with sensitive and excellent nursing care. And to Kathy Malloch my professional partner, my thanks for her friendship, talent, intellect, and commitment to what is best for those we serve. My thanks to my mother Margaret Black who still, after 12 children, 33 grandchildren, and 17 great-grandchildren and a lifetime of giving, has the energy to encourage the best in her firstborn. To all my professional colleagues, I thank you for your courage, caring, and encouragement to me and all nurses in meeting the challenges of caring for others, regardless of how the world changes before them.

Tim Porter-O'Grady

C H A P T E R
1

Making Sense of Transformation: Quantum Realities in a New Age

CHAPTER OBJECTIVES:

Upon completion of this chapter, the reader will:

1. Make sense of complexity concepts as applied to health organizations.

2. Translate complexity notions into leadership processes.

3. Apply concepts of quantum and complexity thinking into decision making, practice roles, and organizational realities.

INTRODUCTION

The cycle of change seems to have quickened and intensified. The problem with current change is twofold. First, the pace of change has quickened so much that it is difficult to keep up, and second, the changes themselves are filled with so many other changes and increasing levels of complexity that they are difficult to understand. People are finding change challenging and difficult to cope with.

The leader's role is directed toward understanding the complexity of change and translating it in a manner that can be understood by those upon whom it impacts. First, however, the leader must find her or his own meaning imbedded in the change, to translate it from a personal perspective with both passion and coherence. Given its current complexities, a different understanding regarding change and its function in the world is unfolding. In today's world, driven by increasing technology, globalization, fiber optic connectedness, and the machinations of complexity science, the leader has much to contend with in translating realities into the common work experience of those he or she leads.

Chaos and complexity as a systems dynamic address elements of the universe as they affect all living systems. As we leave the industrial age, with all that implies, we leave an age that was defined more by the mechanistic elements of function and relationship than by its relational elements. In the sociotechnical age, the understanding of reality operates on a much broader and significantly different premise. Much of the structures, format, and activities of the industrial frame were defined by

> ### Gem
>
> Change never begins nor does it end—it is the fundamental reality of the universe. People don't start to change or stop changing. Change simply *is*!

> ### Newtonian-Age Characteristics
>
> - Reductionistic
> - Vertical
> - Mechanical
> - Hierarchial
> - Compartmental
> - Whole as the sum of its parts

Newtonian realities. Isaac Newton saw the universe as a great machine. Deeper and richer research since then has indicated that the universe, instead of being a great machine, is an even greater set of intersections and relationships. Instead of understanding the universe and its systems and subsystems as a great machine viewed independently, compartmentally, and discretely, the universe can now be understood as something wider ranging and more intensely related than previous Newtonian-based science and research indicated.

Quantum or complexity science is a group of theoretical constructs that look at the universe and its elements as complex adaptive systems. Quantum science seeks the relationship between and among all things and attempts to define the nature of that relationship and its action and impact on all life experiences. Because of the intensity of relationships intersecting between multiple disciplines, questions of complexity are not simple, nor are they easy to answer. Although still in its infancy, complexity science is beginning to provide a broader base of understanding for the actions and intersections of life everywhere in the universe. From the broadest frames of reference to the narrowest and most minute elements, complexity and quantum science looks for themes and the intersections between them.

Quantum science looks at change: how it works, what it means, from where it moves, and to where it is going. Quantum science is actively interested in adaptation, integration, interaction, probability and prediction, and the continuous dynamics of movement.

UNDERSTANDING COMPLEXITY

The leader must know how to incorporate into her or his understanding of leadership this application of multifocal complexity. Furthermore, a leader must apply these notions of quantum reality and complexity to the leadership role and workplace interactions. Within quantum reality, it is increasingly understood that, although the individual is very important, the relationship between and among individuals and their collective relationship to the system is even more critical. The ability to integrate group activities, to cross group boundaries, and to see all systems as a fundamental set of relationships is a critical skill set for the contemporary manager. This leader must reflect an understanding of the independent and interdependent activities that are necessary to create effectiveness and sustainability in systems.

Rather than exhibit unilateral control, this leader recognizes that control must be distributed across the system. This distribution is entirely dependent upon the work, accountability, the authority necessary to undertake the work, and expectations for performance. The leader also recognizes that there must be a goodness of fit between context, content, and outcome. Great change is achieved through small and successful increments of change that when aggregated lend themselves well to the success of greater and broader change. This kind of change is nonlinear and does not represent many past strategies that have been used to undertake change. The quantum leader knows that the relationship between the expenditure of energy or the input of work may not always relate to the breadth and depth of the output. In short, the vagaries associated with work may have little to do with how much work one does, but rather have more to do with the intensity of fit between the activity, the intent, and the outcome. Clearly, the leader must have a new understanding of this complex and dynamic relationship between workers and work.

The nonlinearity of complex adaptive systems tends to favor continuous and dynamic innovation and creativity over stability, a strict format,

---

Quantum-Age Characteristics

- Multilateral
- Multidirectional
- Relational
- Interacting
- Intersecting
- Integrating

Newtonian Conflict

Frank was busy trying to sort out the organizational chart for the hospital. He felt that if he could get people configured on the chart in the right manner, efficiency would result. Alignment of related jobs and responsibilities with the right department was key here. Yet, he was finding it difficult to create such alignments because different relationships needed to emerge at different times and with changing players. Such structuring worked well with large chunks of the organization, but it was problematic when he got to more functional levels of the system. Relationships were fluid and ever changing, depending on the circumstances, and alignments needed to be more fluid. The organizational chart with its hard lines and boxes didn't seem to address that everyday reality.

and unchanging structure. The notion of "attractors" is important in quantum systems. In the Newtonian model, the notion of attractor relates to instantaneous rest patterns or regions, such as the rest moment of a pendulum on a clock. Attractors tend to draw specific energy to them. They are also where the systems action or pattern is energized and bounded. This concept is important because rather than looking at barriers to action, process, or change, the leader begins to look at the inherent energy of the system and asks how to act in concert with it.

Overcoming the machine metaphor in leadership is tricky work. The notion of "machine" is so intensely tied to all our leadership experiences and models that it will be difficult to shift from them. The leader may often find that dependence on the machine model of organization, relationship, or interaction is an impediment to undertaking a more effective leadership role in a quantum format. Combining micro and macro concepts will be equally important.

Emerging science related to the human genome is a classic example of the growing importance of microbiological studies in the future management of disease. On the other hand, human macroevolutionary dynamics have had a tremendous impact on the multiplication and adaptation of the human species. Both of these forms of transformation, micro and macro, have equal importance in understanding health care, and exercising the role of a health service provider requires the ability to embrace both.

For the leader there are important skills that are necessary for applying complexity principles in the expression of the leadership role. In an excellent work outlining the application of complexity theory to health care, called *EdgeWare* (Zimmerman, Lindberg, and Plsek, 1998), the authors enumerate nine basic principles that influence the leader's role in health care. Each one of these principles forms a firm foundation upon which to both conceive and unfold the quantum role of leader. Using these nine principles as a frame, we have explored them with our own unique quantum perspective.

Principle 1.

The leader looks at every activity in the organization through the eyes of quantum systems.

The leader has a great deal of work to do to overcome the existing structures and models of organization in her or his work setting. The "machine" metaphor has been inculcated in both the design and restructuring of clinical work. In quantum thinking, the leader is fully aware that the compartmentalization and vertical orientation of the organization is not adequate for the work being done there.

Clinical work requires strong levels and processes of integration and horizontal relationships. Because of the needs of patients and the clinical activities of the organization, it is critical for interaction and communication to be facilitated across the system. Most health systems, however, are designed to be more vertically integrated than horizontally linked. Although many clinical activities are linked, much of the organizational structures within which they unfold are not connected in the same way. In effective health-care systems, linkages, integration, and interface of clinical and support activities operate continuously and dynamically throughout the organization. The leader, therefore, is continually struggling to accommodate this reality, and sometimes leaders must focus on overcoming the organizational impediments to accomplishing the leader's work and the work of those who provide care.

Many existing Newtonian systems reflect a high need for control. However, clinical providers need great latitude for individual and collec-

---

Kaleidoscope

An easy way to "see" complexity is through the lens of a kaleidoscope. The interfacing and interweaving elements of the constantly changing intersection of parts that continuously "dance" together as they mold new shapes and configurations best represent the components and wholeness of complexity. What is important in viewing the kaleidoscope is the requirement of movement and intersections. Both are necessary for the unending formation of new forms and the unlimited arrangement of possible configurations and relationships in the ever-changing shapes. What a powerful tool for seeing quantum visions.

Creativity over Stability

In the quantum world, stability is a synonym for death. Stability means no movement, which is synonymous with a dead system. Think of how many people and organizations "lust" for the peace and safety of stability in a universe that does everything it can to "upset" the stable and create the conditions for movement and change.

Stability Signposts

- Policy
- Procedure
- Ritual
- Routines
- Org. charts
- Titles & positions

Quantum Leader Characteristics

- Fluid
- Flexible
- Mobile
- Reflects synthesis
- Works from the "whole"
- Coordinates the "intersection"

Quantum Control

So much of management is historically about control. In the quantum world, control is not an issue, change is. Everything is in constant movement, shifting and becoming. The wise leader recognizes that the role of leadership is in managing the relationship of people to the constant movement of the dynamic of change. It is in managing people's response to this constant movement that the leader can ensure creativity, innovation, and relevance remain the fundamental core of all work.

Forces Acting on Work

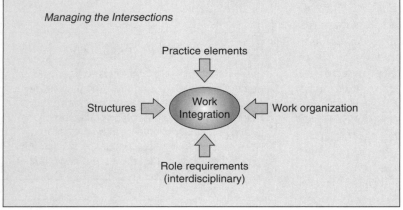

Managing the Intersections

Gem

Leaders recognize that their relationship is with the whole system, not with the department with which they are frequently aligned. Leaders manage their services by bringing their unique service perspective to the whole system and linking and integrating it with other perspectives in order to address the needs of the whole.

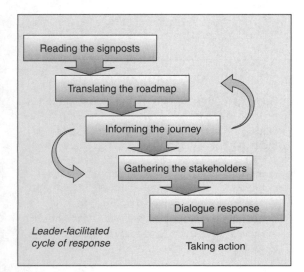

Leader-facilitated cycle of response

tive integration, information, and relationships in the exercise of their clinical work. The leader recognizes this and makes sure that all clinical systems and structures are able to support a more dynamic and interactive frame of reference.

The clinical work of health care is a complex mosaic of intersections and collective activities that requires heavy emphasis on relationship building, communication networks, and well-coordinated interfaces between professionals and structures in the workplace. This is the central focus of the leader's organizing work. Yet, the leader also works to see the hidden intersections and connections in all relationships and where they exist in all organizational and human activity. The leader's focus is predominantly on the intersections and relationships between individuals and functions, support structures and work, organization and clinical activity, and practice and practitioners. This multifocal approach to understanding and applying the leadership role is critical to both effectively seeing the role and applying the necessary skills for facilitating the interactions and confluences to assure that the work is effective and achieves its desired results.

In this set of circumstances the leader begins to conceptualize a change in her or his view of the organization and of the work. The more the leader sees individual activities from the perspective of the whole, noting the common elements embedded in all activity, the more likely the leader will have an accurate perspective of actions and responses necessary to obtain sustainable outcomes. In this way, the leader begins to think about process as a part of structure, structure as embedded in all processes, and both structure and process as fundamental components of obtaining outcomes and creating the conditions for positive relationships and sustainable processes.

Principle 2.

Create the broadest possible vision with any number of variables in which people are free to form and unfold new ways of working and creating.

All systems have a high level of unpredictability embedded in them. This reflects an understanding in complexity and quantum science that simple constructs lead to complex behaviors. The tendency of leadership is to be overly specific and detailed in setting of agendas, developing strategies, or pursuing directions for the organizations and for people's work. In contrast, in quantum reality, over-specifying work and activities interferes with the ability of the system to adapt quickly and easily to changing conditions and circumstances as well as to shifts in work and projects. Indeed, as projects and work unfold, the work itself changes. Doing the work acts as a catalyst for future changes that can only be anticipated as the work unfolds. In this case, experience itself changes the conditions and circumstances of the work. Systems are continually flexible, adaptable, and inherently innovative if allowed to unfold in unpredictable and uncertain ways. The leader must be aware of this confluence of interactions and forces as profound and essential part of unfolding goals and objectives as well as project outcomes.

The leader must be aware that innovation and creation at work respond specifically to environmental and contextual forces. These forces influence much of the contents of programs and projects. The leader must become a good "signpost reader," aware of the environmental and conditional circumstances operating and influencing the conditions and activities of work. Any change in the payment structure for health-care services automatically creates a change in the emphasis, content, and character of those services. A change in social policy regarding confidentiality, for example, has a direct impact on the design, implementation, and management of clinical and business information systems. A new technological discovery in the practice or clinical service creates a new technique and methodology for clinical intervention, changing the mechanism for intervention, the way in which patients are cared for, the way in which processes are paid for, and the supporting infrastructure related to delivering the new service.

What is also helpful for the manager is to recognize the virtuality of complexity and its embeddedness in every level and component of human dynamics and life activity. Processes and interactions are dynamic, not completely dependent on any one function or structural element in the organization. In fact, much of this action goes on out of view, almost at the level of the unconscious, forcing the leader to be aware of the dynamics operating in a higher level than that which is immediately visible. The leader must look at means, threads, or even pictures moving across the backdrop of activity that are clear indicators of process and progress. These indicators may even be activities themselves. In this set of circumstances, the leader is looking for the connections, the points of convergence between efforts and activities, and is attempting to identify the "noise" that indicates they are not working well together or that the confluence of forces are not merging in a way that will create the conditions for integration, operation, and practice, or functional success.

It is also wise for the leader to recognize that a good vision, set of objectives, or focus can lead to a broad base of related effective and essential activities. For example, taking on a new diagnostic technology can have considerable impact across the system. If the diagnostic technology provides an opportunity to diagnose the potential for disease early on, it may eliminate or limit the use of technology currently employed that addresses the same disease when discovered later. The new technology changes or limits the need for and application of technology that may historically have been a source of great service and revenue for the organization. The implication is that the choice of new technology has a broader impact on the effectiveness and focus of the system than simply the individual diagnostic activity of the technology itself. This example is a small indicator of the effect that specific choices might have on other activities in the organization. The leader is always aware of this and is continuously looking at the broader-based implications related to any unilateral, simple, or focus set of choices.

In creating a vision, it is important for the leader to recognize that a simple, broader-based vision may itself transform all the functions and activities in an organization. If, for example, a clinical organization's vision changes from providing good high-quality **bed-based** services to providing equally high-quality **outpatient and ambulatory care**

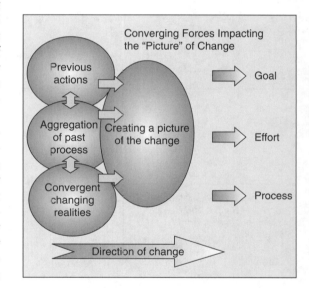

Dynamic Processes

Leaders and staff often conclude that there is an end to particular effort or work process. Leader must take on a new mantle of thinking about beginnings and endings. In quantum change, all process is dynamic and continuous; it neither begins or ends. The leader is continuously engaged in interacting with the constant ebb and flow of all process. The good leaders simply ascertain at what place in the flow specific processes unfold and how those activities lead to the goals being sought.

Converging Forces Impacting the "Picture" of Change

Previous actions

Aggregation of past process

Creating a picture of the change

Convergent changing realities

Goal

Effort

Process

Direction of change

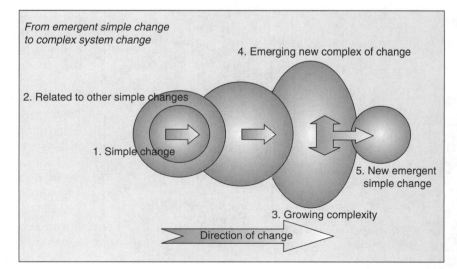

From emergent simple change to complex system change

4. Emerging new complex of change

2. Related to other simple changes

1. Simple change

5. New emergent simple change

3. Growing complexity

Direction of change

services, implications will be considerable regarding the organizational infrastructure, support systems, their priorities, capital planning activities, and financial and revenue considerations. In fact, each and every one of these functional elements will be transformed in ways that are significant for both the viability and the future success of the organization. Here, a simple change in a broadly delineated vision creates complex changes across the system. This holds true with almost any undertaking related to setting visions or goals at any level of the organization.

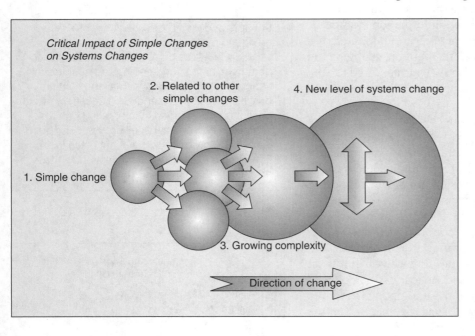

Critical Impact of Simple Changes on Systems Changes

1. Simple change

2. Related to other simple changes

3. Growing complexity

4. New level of systems change

Direction of change

What is critical for the manager and leader, at any level of the organization, is their reflection of the global impact of simple changes in goals, direction, or priorities at any place in the system. These changes, regardless of where they occur, can have broader-based implications for any and all other parts of the system. It is important for the leader to realize that, regardless at what level of leadership he or she operates, he or she has considerable impact on the organization as a whole when making decisions, regardless at what level of the system these decisions are made. In quantum complexity, decisions made at any place in the system can have tremendous implications and impact on decisions and activities unfolding at any other place in the system. While this should not be a frightening consideration, it should be a sobering realization with regard to the implications and impact of decisions that occur at a unit level or any organizational level within the human work system.

Principle 3.

Create a balance between structural and mechanical formality and relational and intersectional dynamics, recognizing the contribution of each to the other and of both to the whole.

There clearly is always the need for structural formation in undertaking and functioning in human organizations. However, what is important to recognize here is that structural formats are tools that give form and discipline to the far more variable and dynamic processes associated with human action. The leader must recognize that balance needs to be obtained between structural elements in the organization and the dynamic elements of human action.

The relationship between structure and human dynamics is not constant or rigid. Additionally, one is not an outflow of the other. What occurs in any given point in time is a continuous "dance" between structure and human action to changes in its cadence, outflow, interaction, and music as the relationship unfolds. The leader maintains a high level of awareness regarding the nature and content of the interaction between structure and human dynamics at any given point.

What often occurs in the dance between structure and action are changes in circumstances, conditions, and external forces in the environment that create a set of new conditions. These conditions now change the circumstances or the

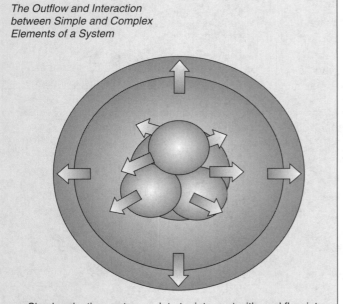

The Outflow and Interaction between Simple and Complex Elements of a System

Simple adapting systems relate to, intersect with, and flow into other simple systems and, when aggregated, create broader, more complex systems in a continuous and dynamic "dance" between them.

context influencing the dance between structure, process, and the relationships of work. The leader in this set of circumstances looks carefully at the mix of these influences and forces and what it says about appropriate action or response at any given moment. The environmental and contextual indicators related to the immediate situation provide more information than a simple assessment of the current situation or activities. Here the leader asks what they are indicating with regard to where the organization is within their context and what signposts are revealed with regard to appropriate response and specific direction. Through reading these contextual factors well, the leader can see and read a better and more appropriate response with regard to direction, priorities, and action choices.

While the leader must maintain appropriate attention to building good supporting infrastructure, he or she must also be aware of the re-

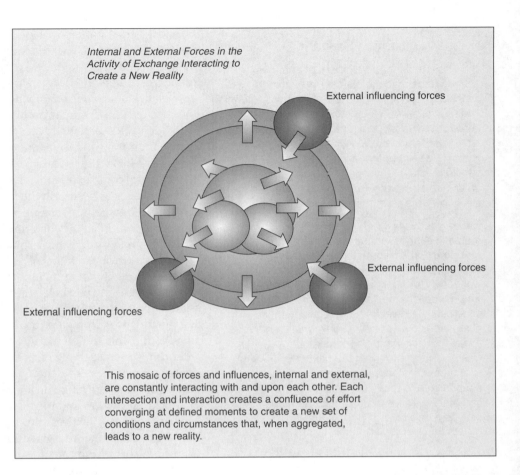

Internal and External Forces in the Activity of Exchange Interacting to Create a New Reality

External influencing forces

External influencing forces

External influencing forces

This mosaic of forces and influences, internal and external, are constantly interacting with and upon each other. Each intersection and interaction creates a confluence of effort converging at defined moments to create a new set of conditions and circumstances that, when aggregated, leads to a new reality.

lationship and confluence of forces that are always indicators of any change moment. Those forces provide information regarding the dynamics of the journey, the elements of change, and the ascending priorities at any given moment that indicate a need for different strategies, a change in direction, or the establishment of new priorities or processes. Structure is modified by the dynamic of the dance of change. The leader recognizes the need to modify, alter, adjust, or even transform structures in order to make the organization more adaptable and more effective in its response to the demands of a given moment or specified change events.

Historically, the greatest problem for organizations has not been their power or influences or economic significance but instead has been their inability to quickly and nimbly adapt to the subtle and sometimes small changes that can transform their circumstances, their conditions, and ultimately their ability to thrive. The good leader makes sure changes in human dynamics are not sacrificed on the altar of form and structure. To the contrary, structure and format should be disciplined by creativity, innovation, and the organization's ability to quickly adapt and adjust to changes. The leader is vital in facilitating this critical dance and assuring that it unfolds in meaningful ways for people as well as the organization.

Principle 4.

The leader must maintain tension between the chaotic and the orderly in managing information, human dynamics, differences, linkages, and environmental and contextual circumstances.

The core of good leadership is always related to achieving balance between sometimes competing and at other times confluent forces. None of the elements identified here have precedence or priority over the others. Weighting of forces such as information management versus orga-

Quantum Guide

The wise leader is always driven by a relationship focus. This leader constantly seeks to better see and configure the interaction between people, processes, and structures. It is this critical interface between these elements upon which the constant forces of change are acting.

Responding to and adjusting relationships, decisions, and actions within the context of people, processes, and structures disciplines the activity of the leader and keeps leadership action focused on the dynamics that lead to sustainable systems change.

Gem

Absolute stability in quantum awareness is a synonym for death. The persons and organizations that fail to continuously adapt and grow are doomed to die. For the leader, it is important to translate this message to all people in the organization: "adapt or die." In this set of circumstances, all work is change and change is the work. This message is the centerpiece of good leadership and the requisite in all leadership performance.

Quantum Scenario

Jim was in a quandary: Important changes needed to be made in his department, and staff was holding on desperately to past rituals and routines. Jim needed to create a set of circumstances that would make it no longer "safe" for them to remain with their past practices. He was concerned with whether he should create a "critical event" by undertaking an immediate change or help them slowly transition toward a change in behavior.

Jim decided in favor of an immediate and dramatic change, creating sufficient chaos to make past practices no longer tenable and forcing the staff to confront the demand for work change. Jim knew that this approach would create immediate reaction and significant "noise." However, he recognized that chaos and noise are essential constituents of all meaningful change and that, as a leader, it was not his role to avoid the pain of immediate change but, instead, to help staff with their adaptation and the development of new tools and processes that would help them adjust to new ways of working.

nizational structural control is not the point of good leadership. Each component of human activity is required in order to effectively coordinate, maintain, and integrate the systems response to the demand for movement and change. The leader should be able to determine the appropriate balance of activities and action at any given time in relationship to the demands on the organization for action or for change.

Biological researchers reveal that absolute patterns of regularity are critical indicators of decline and even death. A certain amount of chaos is required for all life processes to operate effectively. The biological and the universal complex adaptive systems require a certain amount of chaos in their processes to sustain the presence of life. The struggle here is between the degree of chaos necessary to sustain life and the point of chaos beyond which the chaos itself contributes to the decline of life and action. Finding this balance is one of the critical roles of the leader.

Analysis provides a frame of reference for looking at what is. However, analysis alone is not sufficient to be able to address all the issues or forces influencing a particular direction or action. It is a mechanical process for looking at structure, form, circumstances, and conditions and drawing judgments with regard to what responses are appropriate. Analysis plays a role only in determining what the focused action should be. In quantum systems, change lies at the core of all life and function. This care of change creates a demand for a much broader and deeper balance of activities that may include analysis but is not limited to it.

A balance of tools and processes is necessary here to understand the broad mosaic of influences and circumstances that is critical to the role of the leader. The leader recognizes information, not as a thing but as a dynamic, which itself indicates the elements of flow and change. Information is like a river flowing through the human experience and through the organizational structure. Every person in the structure requires information in order to adequately and accurately unfold his or her own work. All individuals must be able to get into the river and gather from it the information and tools necessary to adequately unfold their role in conjunction with the roles and processes of others along the river's edge.

This notion of a flowing, dynamic river of information is critical to understanding the application of information in making decisions, undertaking action, producing outcomes, and evaluating effective performance. Recognized as a part of this flow is the understanding that different points along the river of information require different kinds of resources that are available in a changing format. They alter emphasis and even content depending on the need for information and the point at which that data is gathered. It is the complex interplay along the river's flow that brings value to the use of information. Clearly, different people require different information at different points along the information flow. However, once gathered, all the information creates a composite or aggregate of information that in one way or another will speak to the health, the integrity, and the viability of the organization as a whole. The leader acts as in-

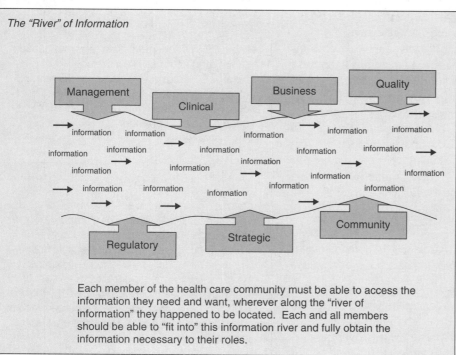

The "River" of Information

Each member of the health care community must be able to access the information they need and want, wherever along the "river of information" they happened to be located. Each and all members should be able to "fit into" this information river and fully obtain the information necessary to their roles.

tegrator, facilitator, and coordinator of the information flow, linked information, and its application as a tool for evaluating the effectiveness and the efficacy of the organization's journey.

While we have used information as one example of the management of flow and of handling change in interacting with chaos, what is important to remember is that the organization, if it is successful, is continuously living on the edge of chaos. Effective, viable, healthy, and alive organizations are those that walk that tightrope between stability and chaos with a tendency to favor the essential chaos embedded in their own necessary changes.

Organizations must be committed to their own change. In order to make those changes there must be in organizations and human systems a connection to the chaos, a willingness to engage its realities, and a process that incorporates the vagaries and uncertainties that chaos brings into the dynamics of planning, strategizing, and acting for the future of the organization. The leader represents this ease with chaos in her or his own role. This person recognizes the essential value of the change dynamic and the chaos that change brings with it and represents well an engagement with and embracing of the realities and elements of chaos. The leader recognizes the levels of functions and structure that are present in the organization. This leader also recognizes that the more the organization is available for the challenges and dynamics of change that foreshadow its future and define its journey, the more successful it will likely become.

Principle 5.

The uncertainty of transformation in change brings with it the necessary engagement of both tension and paradox.

The leader recognizes the need to maintain a specific level of tension in the organization. However, this tension is not related to distress or high levels of painful relationships. The tension embedded in quantum leadership is one that is intentionally maintained between creativity and complexity, on the one hand, and peoples' need for stability and regularity, on the other. The leader recognizes the fundamental need for stability in the organization and incorporates it into the structural elements and components of unfolding work, as well as the relationships necessary to support both the work and the worker. However, the leader does not sacrifice the fundamental tension between order and chaos just to guarantee worker comfort.

A part of sustaining successful activities and the future of the organization is recognizing the tension between current systems functions and operations and the environ-

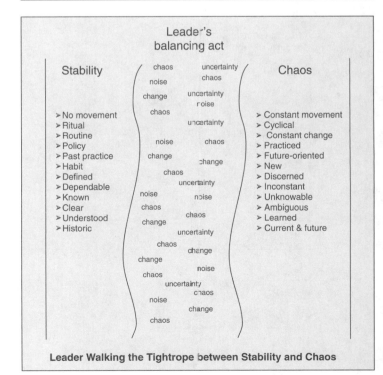

The Tension Tightrope

Change can never occur in the presence of high levels of satisfaction. It is incongruous to expect that people will change those things from which they are enjoying great satisfaction. The leader, then, must manage people at the tension between satisfaction and dissatisfaction. The wise leader recognizes the level of balance in motivating the staff to change between their level of satisfaction and dissatisfaction in the attempt to have staff respond to the need for change. Finding this place of critical tension is challenging, yet is necessary if staff is to engage their own journey of change.

Leader Walking the Tightrope between Stability and Chaos

The Chaotic Paradox

Nancy was struggling with two groups of people in her organization; one eager to undertake the new changes in practice, the other equally as strongly committed to current practices. Nancy knew that changes had to occur; she just wasn't clear exactly what changes were appropriate and what practices should remain the same.

Confronted with this paradox, Nancy decided to get both groups into one room. Using a flip chart, she undertook an intensive dialogue between both groups around the issues and concerns related to the needed change. Using the flip chart to document all thoughts and critical points, Nancy was able to identify the values needed to be retained, the challenges of change, and insights regarding what changes needed to occur and how they might unfold.

By combining both the purveyors of change and those who valued stability, and engaging them both around the need for change. Nancy was able to use paradox as a tool for discernment and built a consensus around a specific direction for change. Furthermore, Nancy was able to engage the stakeholders in the discernment and establishment of their own direction for change.

ment, which is continuously creating the conditions that change current realities. The leader, as the major signpost reader, anticipates the fundamental and essential changes embedded in all movement in human systems. That individual has the responsibility for communicating the movement of change, the impact of that movement on current functions, and the need to prepare for the very next thing. In this, the leader manages the timing, processing, and case for change in a way that balances the stability and integrity of people in the organization with the growing demand for change in the way of doing business.

In dealing with the continuous dynamics of change, the leader learns to master paradox as a way of moving change. The leader recognizes the essential paradox between the fundamental need for stability and the equally fundamental drive for adaptation and change. In managing these realities, the leader uses paradox as a tool for making change. For example, the leader might suggest to a group most reluctant to change how they might maintain their stability and order by radically altering their work processes as a way of ensuring that stability. Clearly, this makes little sense, but it does challenge people to use existing notions and concepts as a vehicle for addressing specific required adaptations and changes.

In living comfortably with paradox, the leader must be willing to raise paradoxical questions as a part of unfolding her or his role in guiding people to undertake essential change. Furthermore, the leader must inculcate in her or his own personal behavior the willingness to live with paradox. The leader asks her- or himself questions about leading and how that might be undertaken without providing control and order as a framework for leadership. How does the leader direct change without initiating that direction her- or himself? How does the leader integrate acceptance of essential change and change activities by modeling acceptance within the context of the leader's role?

The leader creates the conditions and circumstances in which paradox is a part of problem solving and change making. For example, the leader might gather complex groups together with highly divergent opinions in an effort to create sufficient diversity to make any one solution or points of view untenable. The paradox is used as a frame of reference for helping people identify and address essential change. Using the need for stability can form a foundation upon which paradoxical, radical, and significant change can be undertaken in the workers' efforts to maintain their stability and good order. Such processes call the leader to not only embrace the need for paradox but also use paradox as a tool for challenge and change.

Principle 6.

Ambiguity and uncertainty are fundamental conditions for effective change: you don't have to be sure to be successful.

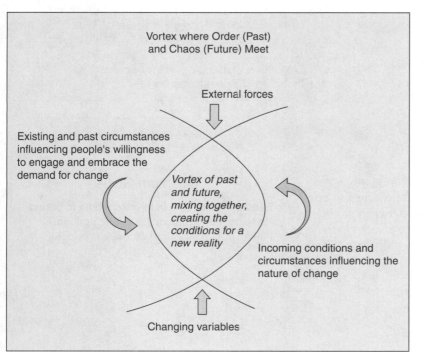

Vortex where Order (Past) and Chaos (Future) Meet

External forces

Existing and past circumstances influencing people's willingness to engage and embrace the demand for change

Vortex of past and future, mixing together, creating the conditions for a new reality

Incoming conditions and circumstances influencing the nature of change

Changing variables

Evolution, heredity, and adaptation are all rife with examples of how uncertainty is essential for the ability to thrive. Indeed, without the necessary diversity and uncertainty of species and the highly variegated environmental conditions of the Earth, there would not have been sufficient differentiation to support life as we know it. Uncertainty is an essential constituent of all adaptation.

Organizations have difficulty with uncertainty. The mechanical foundations of organizational structure and activity exist to remove as much uncertainty as possible from the conditions and circumstances of organizational behavior. By so doing, these organizations contribute to their own lack of adaptation and ability to thrive. One of the fundamental roles of the leader is to assure the organization does not become so enamored of its stability, form, and function that it fails to be aware of the fundamental need to shift and adapt all processes, reflecting the contextual changes that are driving it to thrive in a new or emerging reality.

The leader is constantly aware of the environmental forces and external influences that are creating the conditions for change within organizations. Indeed, the leader's role is to translate the fundamental forces of change into the language of the organization so that its people are continually aware of the action of these forces and their lives. These conditions create the uncertainty that is so much a part of life's experience. It is not that uncertainty is untenable or inappropriate; it is more that uncertainty is frequently ignored, as organizations concentrate more on their function and the stability they so desperately seek.

The leader always lives at the point of uncertainty. In fact, the leader is often a boundary walker, looking down at the issues, concerns, and actions of the organization from its "balcony." From this perspective, the leader begins to gain a better insight of the broad diversity of forces that act in concert to create the conditions for successful change. Nevertheless, the leader knows that no one choice or action unilaterally drives effectiveness or success.

In staying on the fringes of the organization, the leader avoids the temptation to become absolute, certain, and specifically clear about the single most correct action. In fact, good leaders tend to favor experimentation and innovative processes. This tries a number of different approaches to one solution and is a mechanism for finding the best fit between selected processes and an effective outcome. This availability to a variety of approaches and solutions provides a better frame of reference for focusing on those mechanisms that span the possibility of being more successful than simply strategizing, deciding, and directing a solution based on consensus or unilateral decision making

The good leader clearly defines the frame of reference, constructs, or conditions that relate to a solution. But what this leader does not do is find a specific single response or action that will be necessary to a situation's resolution. Instead, the leader gathers individuals around various solutions with the intent of finding in each of them those elements or processes that might lend themselves to addressing an issue or concern in a more meaningful way. Through this availability, or process, or experimentation, or innovation, the leader increases the possibilities of good choice and extends that availability to a variety of elements that may impart a sustainable solution or a whole new set of processes to better advantage the organization and its work.

Gem

Certainty can never be obtained to a sufficient enough degree to eliminate ambiguity. Uncertainty will always be a condition influencing human judgment and decision making. The leader will never have sufficient information or data upon which to know with absolute certitude what choices are right. Information can indicate factors influencing decision making and, when aggregated, can indicate the appropriate direction for choice. However, judgment must still be rendered, risk faced, uncertainty confronted, and action taken. That is the work of leadership.

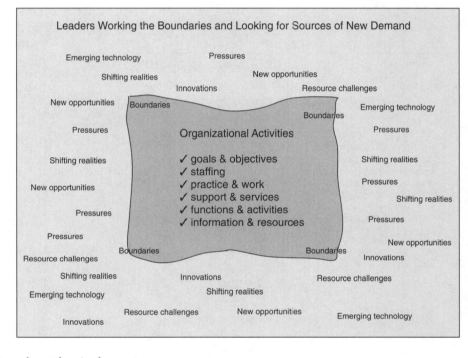

Leaders Working the Boundaries and Looking for Sources of New Demand

Quantum Guide

Leaders make time in their schedule to periodically go to the "balcony." Distancing themselves from their own role and workplace, leaders go far enough away to broadly scan the environment, conditions, and circumstances that affect the lives of people and their organization. This is an essential role of the leader if the leader is not to be drawn into a narrow frame of reference for experiencing change and shifts in roles and performance. The leader is then better able to return to the staff and translate accurately to them the conditions and characteristics of the broader journey. This brings a deeper understanding to their own work experience and acknowledges their particular contributions to the organization's success as a citizen journeying in a larger world.

Formal and Informal Communication Networks

Formal communication structure

- Information system
- Management system
- Clinical infrastructure
- Documentation system
- Business processes
- Telecommunication network

Gossip

Support services network

Workplace dialogue

Secretaries' network

Lunch conversation

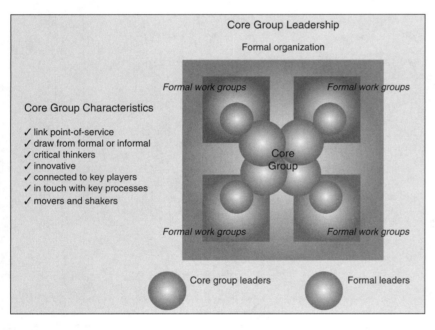

Core Group Leadership

Formal organization

Formal work groups

Formal work groups

Core Group Characteristics

✓ link point-of-service
✓ draw from formal or informal
✓ critical thinkers
✓ innovative
✓ connected to key players
✓ in touch with key processes
✓ movers and shakers

Core Group

Formal work groups

Formal work groups

Core group leaders

Formal leaders

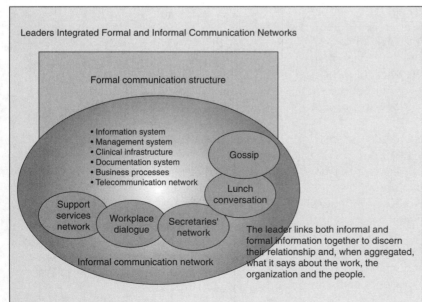

Leaders Integrated Formal and Informal Communication Networks

Formal communication structure

- Information system
- Management system
- Clinical infrastructure
- Documentation system
- Business processes
- Telecommunication network

Gossip

Lunch conversation

Support services network

Workplace dialogue

Secretaries' network

The leader links both informal and formal information together to discern their relationship and, when aggregated, what it says about the work, the organization and the people.

Informal communication network

Principle 7.

The informal organizational networks are critical to an organization's success, as are the formal networks.

Leaders intuitively know that the informal communication and action network of organizations and systems are highly effective tools of communication and information generation. However, this is often not formalized into the ongoing operational reality of the organization. In short, these informal networks are looked at as anomalous, rather than as normative operating processes of human dynamic systems. In formal networks, gossip, story sharing, personal life experiences, and so forth are all a part of the essential constituents of the communication system. Often these informal networks or informal groups of individuals have a greater significance to the effectiveness of the work of the system than do the formal structures and communication networks.

It is perhaps in these informal or shadow networks that much of the creativity and innovation of the organization is located. Indeed, Art Kleiner's new research on core group theory (2004) indicates that many of these powerful individuals and groups are not located within the formal organizational and leadership structure. Yet these individuals and groups have a huge significance with regard to the organization's effectiveness and creativity. Located throughout the system, these core individuals and groups often form informal networks where ideas, notions, innovations, and significant changes are discussed. Any number of stories have been told with regard to how creative and innovative processes have unfolded, not from the ordinary and usual format and structures of the organization, but rather from the serendipitous actions and activities of individuals and groups having gathered informally for purposes other than those defined by work. The leader accommodates this reality and recognizes that through informal networks much creativity and innovation upon which the future of the organization depends gets discussed in a safe context.

Leaders not only value these informal networks, they use them. The good leader tries to access and maintain relationships with some of the better-known components of the informal networks, such as secretaries, unit clerks, housekeeping, and security services, as well as the wide variety of lunch-time gatherings, where the real issues and concerns of the organization are addressed with a great deal of specificity and clarity and in ways not usually permitted within the normal organizational constructs. This leader recognizes these gatherings as fundamental tools of innovation, creativity, and truth telling that help the organization in its own growth and adaptation as well as its orientation to current reality.

The leader recognizes these informal networks hold opportunities to truly problem solve and obtain ideas and notions that might not otherwise be obtained in the formal system. Because of the complexity and compartmentalization of much of the structures of health care, leaders would be advised to join, indeed, create informal networks that operate outside the formal structure. This will provide access to the highest levels of creativity and diversity and leaders can then better apply ideas generated there to the work and dynamics of the organization.

Principle 8.

The most important part of systems is their intersections: larger systems should be the aggregation of successful smaller systems.

In quantum reality, all systems are aggregations of smaller systems. Smaller systems clump together in a dynamic of interaction and intersections to create larger systems when such clumping provides value and meaning for the smaller systems. This reflects a principle that, regardless of the size of the system, "system-ness" is always present, from the smallest measures of intensity to the largest measures of complexity. Indeed, if one wants to understand a large complex system it is better to look for the simplicity that lies at its center.

If one looks at the Internet, it becomes clear exactly how systems operate. As an individual uses the Internet, he or she creates personal intersections, interfaces, networks, and an information complex based on what he or she seeks to do or to accomplish. An individual system is created that meets the specific needs of that individual. However, to interact with the Internet, individuals access a part of a broader, more complex system within which their unique body of information becomes a part of a larger chain and complex of information and access points. This makes it possible for others to draw from the Internet what they need from it. Continuing this dynamic throughout the whole human community, one can begin to see the narrow simplicity and broad-based complexity of interactions and intersections that make the Internet the complex yet simple system that it truly is.

All of complexity is a result of cross-referencing, crossover, and integration of a broad complex of sometimes unrelated sets of elements or factors that, when aggregated, create increasingly complex organizations. Whether computers, the human body, or even the universe, all their elements make up both simple and complex systems. The notion of advancing between the simple elements and the aggregated impact they have on all elements is a metaphor for understanding complex adaptive systems. For the leader, the only way to truly understand complex systems is to be able to effectively make simple systems work well in themselves and then interface well with other simple systems that are also working well. Through this complex integration of simple effective systems, complex systems are built and sustained. A failure of any one system is ultimately a failure in the entire complexity of the larger system. Here the leader recognizes that assuring the effectiveness of the simple functional system and addressing its successful interface with other systems builds the complex array of intersections necessary to sustain larger systems and

---

Seeing Systems

Leaders see themselves from the perspective of the whole system. All leaders identify themselves with the system as the whole rather than with that part to which they are associated. When leaders only associate themselves with their component of the organization, they frequently fail to act in the best interests of the whole. Indeed, they sometimes sacrifice the interests of the whole system for the needs of their service or department. When this happens, their influence and the impact on the system causes both the system and, in the long term, their own department or service to be compromised. Seeing "system-ness" broadens the perspective of the leader, challenging the leader to act locally as through the viability of the whole system was at stake.

Gem

All systems are in motion. The leader is guiding the system "on the fly." As the system continues to move in a dance with its environment, purpose, and circumstances, the leader is working to maintain and sustain a good fit between the organizational environment, purpose, and work. This continual interchange between each of these elements is the essential condition for thriving. In order to assure that systems and people continue to thrive, the leader never forgets that the leader's essential work is embedded in linking and integrating these forces.

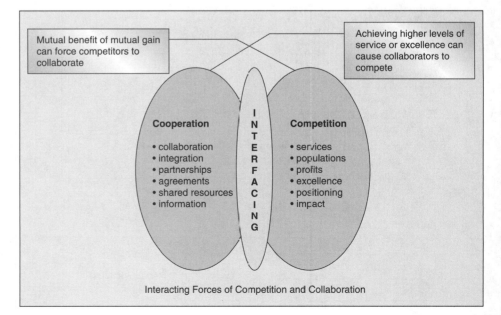

Interacting Forces of Competition and Collaboration

Competing for Quality

Marie and Fred are managers at St. Anywhere's Hospital. They have both been leaders in the hospital for a number of years and have worked diligently to assure the hospital success even in tough times when resources were short. However, although they both cooperated and collaborated extensively in advancing the interests and success of the hospital, they maintained an ongoing competition with regard to measures of clinical quality and service excellence. Marie and Fred constantly competed with each other to see who could achieve the best service and quality scores in the organization. Invariably their departments exchanged measures of excellence as they continue to compete with each other for higher levels of quality.

Marie and Fred present an example of both collaboration and competition expressed in a way that serves as a means to support the system. In this case both collaborated to sustain the success of the hospital, but each also competed over performance measures. Their accomplishments benefited each department, yet at the same time, advanced the interests of the system. Theirs is an example of a continuous and dynamic interplay of the forces of both competition and collaboration.

to assure that simple systems and the larger array of complex systems work in concert to be mutually self-sustaining and life-affirming.

Principle 9.

All creatures both compete and cooperate for resources and for the opportunity to live.

Competition is embedded in the very fabric of life experience in this principle, exhibited at all levels of life from the cellular to the most complex organisms. Competition is a normative and universal experience. Cooperation and mutuality are equally essential to the ability to thrive. Whole communities of creatures at all levels of evolution work in concert to assure their mutual survival.

However, competition is also vital to life. In this paradox, competition is as important to adaptation and sustainability as are mutualism and symbiosis. At all levels of liability in life experience, examples of cooperation between and among species, organisms, environments is as much an example of the activities and structures of life as is competition.

In nature, competition between animals is the most visible representation of the competition built into life. When species prey or feed upon each other in order to sustain life, they are clearly representing competition. Yet at the same time, cooperation between species is also often necessary to mutually support life. For example, African wrens live on the backs of water buffaloes, eating ticks that would otherwise irritate and infect the skin of these animals. In the ocean, smaller fish often accompany unrelated larger fish in order to feed off the creatures that would otherwise infect or endanger the life of larger fish. At all levels of existence, examples of both cooperation and competition are evident in every degree of complexity.

The leader looks for opportunities to visualize complexity and seeks to find the points of competition and cooperation that must exist in equal degrees in order for work to be successful or for the workplace to thrive. In fact, competition may contain within it the seeds of cooperation between competitors when mutual advantage is at stake. The leader may be aware of the need to produce incentives for cooperation even with those with whom he or she may most directly compete. The leader must also incorporate the possibility of forming alliances around specific issues with competitors without sacrificing the other arenas within which the leader would continue to be competitive with another organization.

Neither competition nor cooperation predominates in quantum systems. Whether one prefers to cooperate during competition is an indication of a higher-level issue affecting potential resonance in the system. This does not mean that competitiveness is eliminated as a condition or circumstance of one's life experience; instead, it means that, where cooperation is possible and can advance the integrity of systems and "systemness," it should be the preferred strategy. Here again, however, competitiveness and cooperation are not constant vari-

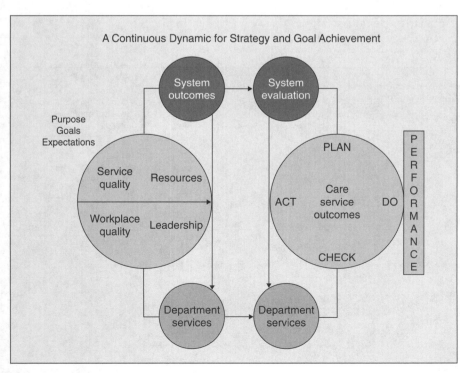

A Continuous Dynamic for Strategy and Goal Achievement

ables. The degree of competitiveness and cooperation may change, depending on the set of circumstances, issues, or frame of reference within which relationships are established. Since these are in themselves a dynamic, they may adjust or shift, ultimately changing the ratio of cooperation to competition. The leader exemplifies an awareness of these changing circumstances and can accommodate them, adjusting the degree of competitiveness and cooperation depending on conditions and circumstances reflected in the relationship between them.

CONCLUSION

Complexity management is simply another tool available to the leader to both understand and apply systems processes in order to effectively guide and lead people and organizations on the journey. Although chaos and complexity models are in their infancy, there is much already available to further our understanding of the application of complexity models in leadership decision making and the design of organizations. Every good leader will develop a growing understanding of the application of complexity and chaos in the exercise of leadership. This new critical concept will have increasing influence over the design and structure of work in the quantum age. Understanding the impact of complexity on decision making, organizational design, relationships, and work and applying it in the exercise of leadership will be essential to the success of the leader in the 21st-century workplace.

Gem

Complexity science calls us to understand the unpredictable, chaotic, and uncertain influences and circumstances that guide the action of all life in the universe. While the leader looks for order and symmetry in the workplace, just beneath the surface lies the chaos and complexity that are the foundations upon which the next order and symmetry will unfold. It is this continuous dance between order and chaos, simplicity and complexity, and leadership and systems that guides the unfolding of the future role of the leader.

REFERENCES

Kleiner, A. (2004). *Who really matters: The core group theory of power, privilege, and success.* New York: Currency.

Zimmerman, B., Lindberg, C., & Plsek, P. (1998). *EdgeWare: Insights from complexity science for health care leaders.* Irving, TX: VHA Publishing.

SCENARIO-BASED FUTURES PLANNING

As the future becomes increasingly important remains basically unclear, it becomes vital to be involved in processes that help organizations and people discern their preferred future. However, rather than predicting the future, it is important to look at the signs (vectors) that, when converged, indicate the pathway or journey to the future, rather than the future itself. Leaders must use a number of creative processes and mechanisms for both gathering stakeholders around their own futures journey and defining the actions and activities that will be necessary to create a preferred future.

Scenario-based approaches define possible conditions and circumstances and the factors that may emerge if those conditions or circumstances unfold. The specific organization or people affected by a given scenario explore the potential responses and actions. Usually three kinds of scenarios are identified: the scenario that emerges if nothing changes, the scenario that exists in the worst possible case, and the scenario that will emerge if all positive factors converge to create an ideal set of conditions or circumstances. Building scenarios is

continues

SCENARIO-BASED FUTURES PLANNING *continued*

like constructing stories reflecting specific and defined elements and components that, when aggregated, give a picture of life within the derived scenario.

Scenario leaders use the following processes in the group's exploration of possible futures:

Brainstorming
Conceptual block busting
Vectoring
Data interpretation
Technology assessment
Financial projecting
Community planning
Demographic shifts
Pattern management
Future search technologies
Consensus decision making

Scenario Exploration

Gather a small group of formal and informal leaders around a single issue, such as patient care, new technology, length of stay, quality or cost control, and so on. Using the single issue as the driver, use the above techniques to "attack" the issue under the umbrella of a different scenario format: whether conditions remain the same, worst-case options, and best-case options. Identify how your world would operate with regard to the specific issue under each one of these scenarios. Remember that current elements, data, circumstances, and conditions provide the backdrop for the scenaric as it unfolds. When scenarios are completed, they can be adjusted with regard to action planning, which will direct the organization to create a preferred future based on the preponderance of the evidence with regard to which scenario appears most appropriate and demands the most specific response.

SCENARIO PLANNING FRAMEWORK

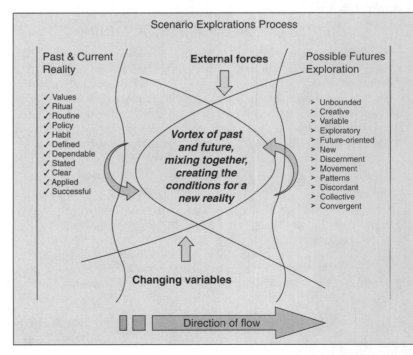

COMPLEXITY CASE STUDY

Sandra has been the clinical manager in critical care for ten years. She has noticed that there has been an increasing level of changes in technology and clinical practice in the past five years. This new technology has created a different way of treating patients and has called clinical providers to adjust the way in which they deliver care for those patients. Because of the new technology, patients are more seriously ill and are now receiving higher levels of complex and intense care. At the same time, the demand to reduce the length of stay has accelerated as costs have increased the the revenue margin has tightened.

Staff have been reasonably responsive to the demand for change. However, there is a good number of staff members who are finding it difficult to let go of past practices and patterns of clinical behavior. At the same time, there is a large number of staff members who are eager to embrace the challenges of new practices and to incorporate them more quickly on the service. Sandra notes that this diversity of behavior is present in the medical staff as well. She's finding it hard to determine whether she needs to take a decisive lead and direct the staff to address these new changes or if she should take the additional time required to engage them in dialogue and group process so that together they might determine the best methods of action. Time is of the essence, yet all must be involved.

A group of the critical care staff have been meeting informally over lunch to talk about some of the issues in the service and to discuss matters of concern with regard to changing practice and new patient care demands. They have come up with many creative suggestions and are eager to begin implementing them as soon as possible. Sandra appreciates their contribution but is beginning to feel as though she's losing control and now is no longer the source of providing direction in her department.

Administration, using a "future search" approach, has developed a new strategic plan and set of goals and objectives for the health system. Each department has fully participated in the development of the strategic process and now must begin to incorporate the strategic goals into the operation and activity of the department. Every department must give evidence of advancing the strategic goals of the organization, a part of which is departmental competition for advancing quality and service excellence. Sandra must begin to build this initiative in her department. She is feeling challenged and is unsure how to manage all of this work and still implement new sets of priorities and actions in her department.

Complexity Case Study Questions

Using quantum examples from the principles outlined in this chapter, review Sandra's leadership case study and respond to the following questions that reflect leadership in a quantum age.

1. What are three elements of complexity that can be identified in Sandra's circumstances?
2. Is there conflict or resonance between the organization's method of creating a vision and direction and Sandra's obligations to do the same in her department?
3. How certain does Sandra need to become about her issues and responses to them before she undertakes action?
4. Does Sandra have issues around controlling information, the content of work, the distribution of power, and the management of personal and institutional anxiety?
5. What are the paradoxes Sandra is now confronting in the course of providing clinical care and doing the business of the department?
6. Sandra must act on multiple levels. What are those multiple circumstances and levels of action that must occur in order for the unit to continue to grow and to thrive?
7. What is the emerging power of the informal system? Has the core group changed the dynamics of leadership and the movement of change?

8. What is the relationship between the larger organization (larger complex system) and the department (smaller complex system), and how is the tension and resonance between them now managed differently?
9. What are the elements of competition and collaboration that are reflected in the departmental goals and staff activities?

Application

Take the same questions and apply them to your own department's concerns or issues. Begin your discussion of your own department's issues by focusing on a particular problem or concern currently confronting the service or the department. In the context of group dialogue use the questions above to explore the issues and concerns. Try to establish a different frame of reference for answering them and a new set of processes for responding to them. Remember, there are no limitations or parameters, so exploration, innovation, and creativity are the tools that should be applied to this group process.

SUGGESTED READINGS

1. Battram, A. (1998). *Navigating complexity.* London and Sterling, VA: The Industrial Society.
2. Goldsmith, M. (2003). *The many facets of leadership.* Upper Saddle River, NJ: Financial Times/Prentice Hall.
3. Griffin, G. S. (1996). *Complexity theory in construction management.* Unpublished doctoral dissertation, Colorado State University.
4. Janssen, M. (2002). *Complexity and ecosystem management: The theory and practice of multi-agent systems.* Cheltenham, UK: Edward Elgar.
5. Lewin, R., & Regine, B. (2000). *The soul at work: Listen, respond, let go: Embracing complexity science for business success.* New York: Simon & Schuster.
6. Lewin, R., & Regine, B. (2001). *Weaving complexity and business: Engaging the soul at work.* New York: Texere.
7. Lissack, M. (2002). *The interaction of complexity and management.* Westport, CT: Quorum Books.
8. Mainzer, K. (2004). *Thinking in complexity: The computational dynamics of matter, mind and mankind* (4th rev. and enl. ed.). New York: Springer.
9. McElroy, M. W. (2003). *The new knowledge management: Complexity, learning, and sustainable innovation.* Boston: KMCI Press.
10. Olson, E. E., & Eoyang, G. H. (2001). *Facilitating organization change: Lessons from complexity science.* San Francisco, CA: Jossey-Bass/Pfeiffer.
11. Ragsdell, G., West, D., & Wilby, J. (2002). *Systems theory and practice in the knowledge age.* New York: Kluwer Academic/Plenum Publishers.
12. Samad, T., & Weyrauch, J. (2000). *Automation, control, and complexity: An integrated approach.* New York: Wiley.

Leading in a New Age

CHAPTER OBJECTIVES:

Upon completion of this chapter, the reader will:

1. Understand the new requisites of leadership.

2. Identify the critical elements of competent clinical leadership.

3. Name the characteristics of "new age" leaders and the changes in the expression of the role.

4. Enumerate the changes in the 21st-century workplace influencing both the work and worker and forming the context for "new age" leadership.

INTRODUCTION: A DIFFERENT AGE

Everything is different. As we leave the industrial age everything about work and leadership is changing. The leader must be aware that older skills and talents gained from experiences in previous learning are newly subject to question. Work now represents a whole different set of values, interactions, and intersections and requires the ability to integrate, coordinate, and facilitate these dramatic changes in work.

The problem of all this change is that much of what leaders have learned in the past for addressing change is no longer adequate for today's emerging demands for leadership. As a result, leaders are often frustrated with a lack of skills to address the changing character of work, and employees are uncomfortable with the quality and content of the work of those who lead them. As a workplace changes, so does the need for leadership. However, in order to lead well, the leader must gain new insights and skills, change the talents and abilities acquired over a lifetime of experience, and adapt and adopt new behaviors and patterns of leadership to better reflect the context for work in today's environment.

Along with significant technological innovations, changes in communication, and the globalization of work, leaders also must adjust to instant communication, unbounded relationships, the globalization of economics, a shifting political landscape, high-tech clinical processes,

> ### Gem
> It's a new world for organizations. No longer can the old institutional models of work and workplace govern how and what people do. It is now time to rethink the very foundations of work.

> ### New Age Characteristics
> - Mobile
> - Portable
> - Fast
> - Fluid
> - Flexible
> - Systems-driven
> - Digital
> - Relational

A Meaning for Work

The role of the leader is to provide a context for meaning. Workers need to get back in touch with the "why" of their work: the reason they do what they do. Work always changes, as it should. What should remain constant, however, is the value of the work and the meaning each individual brings to it. This meaning gives them their reason for doing work and their desire to keep growing and expanding their skill and their effort.

Change Is Forever

Change never changes! Leaders must understand that change is the work and will be the single constant in all human activity. Embracing this reality is the essential cornerstone to effective leadership. It informs the work of the leader and calls on leaders to incorporate the reality of constant change into all work relationships and action. Staff must know that they cannot stop change, nor slow it, or even alter it. They can only respond to it, giving it the form it will take, and addressing the impact it will express.

Chaos & Calm

Chaos does not always mean "noise." Calm in the fact of chaos exhibits a basic understanding of the work of chaos in changing our frame of reference, our direction, or our activity. Chaos serves a purpose and acts to challenge our insights and sensibilities, calling us to a new way of seeing and being.

Industrial Age Infrastructure

- mechanical
- functional
- structured
- reductionistic
- vertical
- compartmental

knowledge management, and a host of other challenging and daunting changes in the way in which human beings relate and interact together. All this has a dramatic impact on the ability of the leader to provide meaning, value, and a clear direction within the context of the 21st century.

Simply dealing with the context of leadership and the drama of new emerging work realities can frequently be overwhelming for leaders. Indeed, it is overwhelming for organizations. The pace of change and the demands of that pace are so challenging that it appears almost beyond human competence to be able to address these changes in a meaningful way. As a result, leaders and those they lead must now live more comfortably in the ambiguity and the challenges of permanent change, which is often called "permanent whitewater."

This notion of continuous and endless change as a dynamic for work is an important concept upon which the leader must build. Construction of new leadership must occur within the context of emerging new frames of reference for work. The leader must recognize that change is itself the work. Understanding the notion of change as a permanent human condition, rather than as a set of circumstances that can be managed and manipulated, is an important first step. They must conceive change as a permanent, contextual and conditional circumstance of all work. Recent research on complexity indicates that change is the normative condition of the universe. Human beings do not create or make change; instead, they give change its form, the way in which change can unfold in realistic stages, applying meaning to the human experience. Change is a lived experience, forever "dancing" across the consciousness on the landscape of human experience.

The leader must engage change with the expectation that it is a permanent condition. Leaders must exemplify in their own role a constant and continuous engagement of change as a fundamental part of their leadership experience. Within their own behaviors and adaptation, leaders exemplify a living accommodation to the constancy of change. Representing this reality as a personal leadership example and model of engaging change is a critical part of the leader's role in helping others to both understand and adapt to the permanent condition of change.

All people desire some level of stability in their lives. The challenge for the leader exists at the point of tension between personal stability and the ever-evolving dynamic of change. A critical role that change plays in individuals' lives must be facilitated by the leader in a way that assures continuous growth for individuals while, at the same time, maintaining the comfort and calm often found in the ritual and routine of human experience. This is a special challenge. Leaders must be able to demonstrate in their personal lives and leadership the engagement with and embracing of change. They must be able, at the same time, to maintain sufficient calm, peacefulness, and adaptability so staff can incorporate those qualities in their own roles as they confront life-changing events. In this way, leaders become conduits for change, instruments that staff can witness and themselves incorporate as an appropriate model of engagement and accommodation to change.

Leading in a Forever Fluid World

Much of the institutional infrastructure of the industrial age represented a more mechanical application of work. As newer models of work emerge, driven by increasingly broad-based technological innovations, entire new constructs and frameworks for work also emerge. Leaders must now conceive of work as a highly fluid and mobile exercise, challenging old notions of fixed and compartmentalized structures and frames. Even the industrial notion of "job" presents a perspective of work that is individualistic, unilateral, nonaligned, and functionally focused. Job descriptions, the tools that have most articulated the content of work, are no longer adequate for defining work. Today, work changes so quickly in its content that identifying it becomes deceptive. Job descriptions no longer address expectations and performance clearly and specifically enough to have any meaning. In fact, the content of work is changing so quickly that codifying it becomes an exercise in futility. Now, instead of job functions, individuals must identify their work within the context of specific roles. Workers must look at their role in light of its intersections, relationships, and work demands. It is these interactions that provide better insight and understanding with regard to the content of work roles and the exercise of work. In short, people must recognize that work's role is better defined by its relationship to others and to outcomes than by any definition of permanent content.

The stable institutions of the 20th-century workplace no longer represent either the framework or the circumstances of work for the 21st-century workplace. The old "bricks and mortar" institutionally fixed settings and structures for work are not the prevailing reality for the form and context of 21st-century work. Fluidity, mobility, the ability to do work at any time, any place across the globe exemplify the contemporary vision of work. Cellular phones, laptop computers, wireless networks, global accessibility; these all reflect changing conditions that challenge our notion of work. Historically, work required a specific time and place and was much more structured and formal and bounded with more clearly delineated parameters. Now work can be performed anywhere on the globe. Workers connect across the globe using contemporary technology, changing the very nature of interaction and communication as well as work performance. As a result, the locus of control for work, decision making, and relationships is now shifting from fixed work sites to highly mobile work processes.

This shift in the locus of control reflects a change in the nature of work, the nature of work relationships, and new intersections between worker and workplace. Leaders must recognize that the worker is becoming increasingly competent in controlling and managing the variables associated with his or her own work. The locus of control for content of work and the relationships necessary to sustain it are moving inexorably from manager to worker. This creates conditions and circumstances that allow the worker to be more self-directed, the work to be more decentralized, and the workplace to be more fluid.

Several new elements emerge as a result of this change that permanently alter the social conditions of work. There's a greater desire and need for workers to have more highly technical skills. There is also a need for the more educated worker, a desire for more technically prepared workers, and a better interface between the unique technical skills of each worker. In this set of circumstances, the leader must align all of these skill sets in a way that advances the outcomes of work. The social challenge embedded in this is the reduction in demand and need for nonskilled or uneducated workers, forever changing the landscape of work. As with everything in a complex world, the interactions and intersections of the work demands creates social and political circumstances that require a change in the infrastructure that supports human activity.

New Leadership, New Expectations

It is clear that traditional, industrial-age skill sets operating in the framework of institutional models of work are no longer sustainable. These work

---

"New Age" Infrastructure

- wholistic
- relational
- synthesis
- multifocal
- multidirectional
- integrated

No Role for Job Descriptions

In a time of great change, the role for job descriptions diminishes considerably. Changes in function, activity, purposes, and goals of work shift so quickly that describing them in job categories no longer suffices. Descriptions and definers of work now require a clearer identification of the purposes and the outcome of work rather than the functions and processes of any work category. More importantly, the confluence of work efforts and the integration of individual roles within a team context is a more important delineation of the characteristics of work than job descriptions can ever provide.

Workers Control the Means of Work

- Local decisions predominate
- Decisions made where they are implemented
- The work is "knowledge" work
- Quality depends on who does the work
- Efficiency requires competent decisions
- Clinical decisions require ownership by clinicians

Command and Control

- centralized
- unilateral
- vertical
- directed
- superordinate
- hierarchical

Shared Decisions

- decentralized
- team-based
- horizontal
- inclusive
- engaging
- accountable
- point-of-service based

models cannot operate successfully in a highly mobile work environment. The globalization of work alters notions and processes such as job descriptions, performance expectations, job compliance, management-driven decision making, and hierarchical structures. The vertical constructs for decision making and the command-and-control structures are no longer the means by which managers can assure the work is appropriately done and outcomes are achieved. This more mechanical notion of the relationship between worker and work as well as worker and workplace can no longer be sustained. The relationship in the new workplace is far more dynamic, interactive, and increasingly interdependent. It is in this developing frame of reference within which the role of the leader must now unfold.

Leaders need to recognize that their role is predominantly transformational as they confront the vagaries of the "new age." It is in this transformational change, especially in its initial stages, that the leader must be able to demonstrate an understanding of the content of change and the impact that change will have on the worker and the workplace. In this first stage, leaders must exemplify a level of frankness and honesty that at times may appear painful and challenging to those who must hear about the radical nature of work changes. Leaders must persuade followers to embrace the imperative of change in their own work and the need for immediate behavioral and role adjustments. Leaders must exemplify that competency is always shifting depending on demand. In order to remain continuously competent, workers must be continually engaged in addressing the content and influences of their own work. As technology creates new means of working and demands on the work itself, workers must shift their emphasis. This is especially critical when one considers the degree of technological shifts and their impact on therapeutic care and treatment of patients and rendering health-care services. Much of the education of the practitioner is now dependent on immediately meeting patients' needs over shorter lengths of stay. As a result, caregivers have less time to render the same kinds of service that they once provided over much longer periods of time. Caregivers must now raise work-related issues about what activities are critical to care, what activities must be left behind, and what new activities are emerging, created by the demand for applying new technology. This new work changes the nature of the relationship between patient and provider. It requires leaders to address the meaning of the change, the content of the activities of work, and the time frames needed for accomplishing the clinical work in a way that is effective, efficient, and meets the needs of the patient. It is the leader's role to make sure that the elements and fundamental circumstances of a change in emphasis and priority are part of the deliberation and decision making of the clinical staff. The leader must help the staff confront those things that are no longer usual and ordinary, including the clinical activities to which they have been accustomed. Often the staff must give over old ways of doing business in order to adapt to new applications and technologies and do this quickly and efficiently.

Adaptation is critical to the staff's ability to succeed. In order to help staff adapt, the leader, constantly living in the potential, anticipates the changes that will affect work and translates those changes in language the staff can understand. Furthermore, the leader helps the staff in applying new concepts and notions of work, by making it safe to risk, experiment, challenge, and evaluate new methods of clinical performance. The leader in this set of circumstances exemplifies in the role an individual commitment to adaptation and change by making risk and experimentation safe and appropriate strategies for organizational and individual adaptation.

Leadership Honesty

- direct
- frank
- disclosing
- open
- vulnerable
- exploratory
- discourse-friendly

Leadership Dishonesty

- secretive
- polarizing
- noninclusive
- exclusive
- controlling
- selective
- incomplete

Gem

There is a new relationship between the patient and the caregiver requiring a new level of honesty about what is or is not going to happen. Caregivers must now realize that they have to reteach the patient what to expect in a different model for service delivery. Remember, much has changed since the patient's last experience, except for the patient's own expectations. These expectations now must be changed to match the current reality for service if patient satisfaction is to ever be achieved.

Adaptation

Fluidity and flexibility are now a requisite of all work. Holding onto past practices and nonrelevant traditions that do not better serve the patient is a failure strategy. The leader must require a new way of both seeing and doing the work and provide a safe context for clinical change. Stoking the expectation for changes in practice is a minimum requirement for good leadership.

Because the leader anticipates the next cycle of change, he or she keeps an eye on the broader frame of reference for all work activities. Leaders look for meaning in change to guide its translation into the lives of workers in a way that can be understood and applied. For example, much health care today requires providers to rethink service delivery and how to make it more portable, fluid, and easy for the patient to access and use. Increasingly, patients are healing in places other than health-care institutions and now require a level of information and access to clinical support that was once available to them from their caregivers when that support was provided directly by caregivers in hospitals. Leaders now must translate this set of circumstances and guide their followers to make decisions about how skills once offered in the institution can now be provided to patients in other settings. This role of "translation" of change is a vital part of the role of the leader, as new concepts and notions of service must be defined and incorporated within the context of the emerging contemporary role of the caregiver.

In inaugurating a new paradigm for work, the leader must emphasize a different set of principles. Delineating a new set of rules for staff, the leader needs to create a different framework and way of thinking for staff that helps everyone understand the emerging new demands for work.

1. *The leader must be able to address the inner resources and wisdom of both leader and follower.* The leader can't know everything about change or the impact of change on work. Good leaders access collective wisdom and utilize it in helping teams adapt and adjust to whole new ways of doing business. Leaders must engage all participants in the system to develop a level of interpersonal competency and contribution that helps the work and learning team find common ground, share mutual and unique competencies, meet the challenge of change together, and develop new patterns of work and relationships. This requires high participant approaches to the application of leadership. In this case, the leader is essentially a "gatherer," making sure the right stakeholders are at the decision-making table with regard to work and its exercise.

   The leader recognizes that no work is essentially independent. All work activities have a level of interdependence that recognizes the impact of anyone's role on all other roles. This essential interdependence requires in the leader a broad competence in applying systems thinking in decision making at all levels. Furthermore, the leader must be able to articulate in the followers' roles his or her own understanding of the impact of individual action on others. Leaders must translate their understanding of collective wisdom and the intersection of all efforts in the roles of each provider. What must result in the workplace is the respect and understanding of the value and importance of the unique contribution of each worker and the collective integration of those contributions in making a substantive difference in the care of patients.

   Leaders represent a deep understanding that all work reflects a mosaic of interfaces that when pulled together act as a "whole" in moving to achieving sustainable outcomes. Reflecting this understanding in the application of the leader's role creates an appreciation in the follower with regard to the value of worker's own efforts. Rather than seeing unilateral action as desirable, this systems reality creates in the worker an understanding that individual action must fit with the collective enterprise. The resulting mosaic of individual actions must substantially link and integrate in a way that ultimately has a meaningful impact on the patients

---

"User-Controlled" Health Care

The system in which most providers were "born" was designed to be provider-driven and controlled. With the introduction of the Internet and "mass-customization," the user is being empowered to control more aspects of choice and action, forever changing the rules governing service and decision making. Users are taking control. The obligation of the provider now is to make sure the user becomes competent in exercising control and to do whatever is necessary to make the user competent.

Building Interdependence

The leader's primary role is to build real and sustaining sense of team. The interdependence now necessary to good service is such that care cannot be successful without team-based commitment to designing a delivering service. The core element of interdependence must be inculcated into all work.

- collaboration
- integration
- consensus-based
- dialogue-driven
- clearly delineated roles
- common goals (negotiated)
- mutuality of function

Creating the Service "Mosaic"

- All roles are linked
- Define the intersections
- Clarify the boundaries
- Define the mutual expectations
- Commonly agreed-upon goals
- Continuous learning and adaptation
- Frame for resolving conflict

served. This wisdom calls all workers to a different level of understanding with regard to the meaning and relationship of individual work versus the work of the team. This realization affects decision making, collaboration, and clinical action at every level of application. It is the leader's role to make sure this reality is constantly before the staff, continually reminding them of this synthesis of activity as a means of integrating and investing staff in the work of the whole.

2. *It is the leader's role to acknowledge the interconnectedness of everyone and everything.* Everything that all people do has some relationship to everything everyone else does.

There is always and everywhere a continuing dynamic and synthesis of activities that ultimately relate to all other activities. This results in a perpetual interface of motion and process acting in concert with the movements and flow of life. One of the cognitive competencies of leadership now is the application of systems thinking to problems and issues, indeed, to the work itself.

Self-management and servant leadership are now essential characteristics influencing the role of the leader. Collective effort doesn't diminish the impact of individual effort, it simply indicates the value of that effort when aggregated with the whole. Leaders are challenged to create much stronger team-based and relationship-driven work systems. The contemporary leader must focus not only on individual performance, but also on the interconnectedness and intersections of performance and the collective products of good work performance.

Individuals can no longer be encouraged to solve problems in isolation. Leaders must actively search for opportunities to build the proper connections, collective creativity, positive human relationships, and the use of intuitive processes for problem solving. The leader uses tools of participation, relationship, and interpersonal interaction. The skilled leader must have well-honed interpersonal and interactional competencies. Not only must this leader be able to express these competencies but he or she must also be able to translate them well for followers, so that they express these competencies in the exercise of their own roles.

The role of the leader must also reflect change in the dynamics of application of the role. Leaders must see themselves as servants to those who do the work, as well as to the organization. This notion of servant leadership creates a different model of the application of the leader role. It calls leaders to see themselves in the context of the service role rather than from the traditional hierarchical position of the manager. Positional considerations for the role are no longer as valuable as relational considerations. In this new context, the application of the leader's role represents a facilitation and access to resources, systems, supports, and information in any way that advances the viability of the work of the staff. While this is not a new concept, it is no longer optional. The expression of the role calls for deeper notions of partnership, collateral relationship, hor-

Creating the Mosaic of Intersecting Action

3. Mosaic grows in complexity

1. All change is related

2. Each element relates to all

4. Mosaics in constant movement (change)

The Servant Leader

- lateral role with the staff
- seeks to support staff decisions
- provides information for staff decisions
- open to staff direction
- uses group process
- facilitates challenging decisions
- advocates for staff leadership

Servant Leader Skills

- vulnerable
- open
- adaptive
- inclusive
- direct and honest
- group dynamic skills
- great role modeling

izontal decision making, and collective problem solving. Here again the leader must exemplify these skills, first in the role of the leader, and through its application create exemplars for the staff so that the same behaviors can be found in staff roles too.

3. *Hierarchies must be deconstructed.* People can no longer only focus on specialized and defined tasks. While efficiency is certainly obtained through specialization and work focus, effectiveness is sustained by recognizing the integration of all activities around a common goal. What hierarchies do support is the differentiation and compartmentalization of work in decision making. What often happens is that flexibility, fluidity, innovation, risk taking, and challenge are designed out of responsive creative action. The hierarchical configuration of systems and work processes creates a significant management structure and legitimizes that structure to undertake decision making and evaluation of work and performance.

Often an organization's departments that could be identified as servant structures, such as finance, human resources, and information systems, become decision points guiding and directing organizational decision making in ways that are ultimately inappropriate and nonproductive. Rather than playing a servant's role, they provide a primary decision-making role, hijacking legitimate and effective decision making. In the transformative organizational context, those services that most represent the core business of the organization play the predominant decision-making and application role. However, what is required in this set of circumstances is that those departments (such as finance, human resources, and information services) must make sure that these primary decisions are informed by specialized information available in support departments.

Of course, this calls for a whole new way of looking at relationships and roles. These intersections between support and service call for reframing interaction and decision making. A huge reformatting of the structural integration of support and service systems will be required as well to properly configure health-care organizations in a way that focuses on service, quality and value. Indeed, value will only be fully achieved through a massive overhauling of the structure and organization of health care in a way that reorients the operational priorities to better support core services and the obtaining and advancing of clinical and service value. No organization that sacrifices its core "business" has ever survived. How many times have hospitals done that in the past two decades alone? Perhaps, on a more detailed review, the current nursing shortage is a payback for "turfing" nurses out of hospitals during the days of "reengineering," when they were replaced with more functional and less skilled workers. Certainly this is a heavy price to pay, as the complex demands of care today require more resources with a higher level of skill and competence and fewer nurses are available.

Leadership at that time would have required great courage on the part of nurse executives and managers in the face of overwhelming demand from their administrators to cut staff in order to comply with the prevailing cult of reengineering.

It is precisely this disoriented hierarchy that places the clinical decision-making process beneath the financial and operational decision structure, even though these clinical services are the core of the work of the health-care system.

Deconstructing Hierarchies

- Bring decisions to the staff
- Disclose necessary information
- Develop group skills in staff
- Develop shared decision-making processes
- Build staff ownership of issues and solutions
- Have staff confront normal conflict
- Create staff social cohesiveness (celebrating)

Gem

Leader should never allow staff to transfer decisions and accountability for action to the leader. Staff ownership of all issues is critical to accountability, which cannot be sustained if the leader acts for the staff. The leader must never own decisions and actions that belong to the staff and must make sure staff never transfers them out of their own locus of control.

Leadership Courage

Courage is a fundamental skill necessary to all leadership. It is the one thing that can only be demonstrated through the behavior of the leader. There are "signs" that the staff need to see in the leader to indicate he or she acts courageously.

- Does not hold back negative news
- Speaks up in controversies
- Does not fear sharing views
- Is direct with others
- Can express countervailing views
- Does not shy away from noise
- Engages change directly

NEW CORE COMPETENCIES FOR THE HEALTH-CARE LEADER

The leader must be able to evidence the engagements of significant change in his or her own role. While not blinded by past success or limited by it, the new leader must reconceptualize the worldview of the staff and renew a focus on their core values, beliefs, practices, and notions. Indeed, the leader must do that for her- or himself. Health-care leaders must change not only the way they think but also the way they act and how they engage others in decision making and in clinical action.

Therefore, specific competencies that are critical to the unfolding role of the leader include conceptual, participation, interpersonal, and leadership competencies. Each has critical elements that are important to their expression and has a significant impact on the role of staff. The leader must be able to demonstrate facility in the expression of these skills if staff are to be able to perform well within the context of a new work reality.

The expression of management knowledge gives evidence of the mind maps or conceptual schemes that leaders reflect. Leaders create context for others' work. Therefore, the leader must be able to translate concept into reality for staff in a language that they can understand. The leader must create a sort of mind map that becomes for the staff both process and outcome. The use of these leadership mind maps assists in leadership action planning and helping staff through new experiences. Using these mind maps, leaders can help staff rethink and reconceptualize their activities and their work within the context of the new format for that work. Through the stages of development, such as direction setting, decision making, communicating processes, structural design, interpersonal and interdisciplinary interaction, and consensus building, the leader guides the staff to a different and higher level of practice. The leader recognizes that no change is going to occur unless the staff is able to articulate and incorporate it within their own understanding. The leader must not only develop strong conceptual competency but strong translation skills as well.

While mind maps provide a strategic framework for directing action, they can also be limiting. The leader must be constantly aware of the accuracy and timeliness of her or his own conceptions and mental models. Outdated or inaccurate concepts or notions of clinical work or the context of work can prevent concerted and meaningful action. Furthermore, they can limit the leader's ability to identify social and organizational cues, which can lead staff in the wrong direction rather than provide support for them. The leader must remember that critical cues reflect the leader's own ability to see them. Therefore, the leader must constantly check and recheck the mental map that is used for decision making to make sure that it is congruent with the shifts and changes in the context within which work unfolds.

The most important conceptual skill for the leader today is the development of true systems thinking. The systems thinker doesn't simply look at health-care delivery as an organized group of services, compartmentalized and configured to meet patient needs. Instead, the leader sees care delivery as an integrated set of service configurations and interfaces that operate together along a continuum of health and illness to advance the interests of the patient. The leadership role is grounded in accountability and managing core interactions rather than simply operating at the

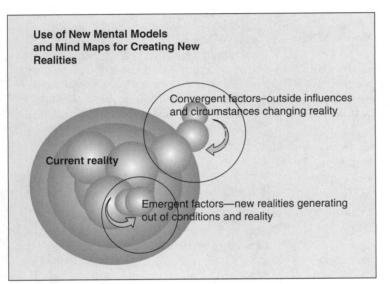

Use of New Mental Models and Mind Maps for Creating New Realities

Convergent factors—outside influences and circumstances changing reality

Current reality

Emergent factors—new realities generating out of conditions and reality level of control. In this case, problems are not seen in isolation from each other but are a necessary part of a larger universe of interactions and intersections that must be addressed. Problems and medication administration or patient care can be looked at, not simply as the fault of an individual but within the context of a system of delivery. This system of delivery is affected by workload, knowledge, resources, workflow, and a set of standards and practices that guide the delivery of medication. The leader sees all these elements in concert and addresses them within the context of one great relationship rather than in iterative and functional segments. The health-care leader recognizes that the whole is greater than the sum of its parts, the power of language and expression reflects the conceptual foundations the leader maintains, and the leader's own ability to translate concept into reality depends fundamentally on his or her relationship with others.

The 21st-century leader struggles with all the confusion and chaos that affects the ability to translate concept into action. In the past, leaders have been taught to equate control with order. We know, however, through quantum thinking that stability is a symptom for death. Innovative and creative environments require equally innovative solutions, which cannot be obtained without confronting the vagaries and noise of instability, chaos, and uncertainty. This level of being overwhelmed is a constant condition in the process of change and is often reflected in followers' reactions. The leader must model an ability to deal with chaos by partnering with it, engaging its energy, and sorting through the information it is attempting to generate with regard to how things are changing. The leader attempts to reap the deep meaning from the chaos and to rescue from the flux and movement of chaos the inherent order, appropriateness, and concerted action that must be taken to continue the movement forward.

Certainty is not required for action. This does not mean that the leader has permission to act without thinking or without verifying the collective wisdom in any given pursuit. However, uncertainty calls the leader to sort through the confluence of forces (the vectoring) to determine what direction is indicated by the convergence of the vectors. In order to do this the leader must exhibit several ways of thinking:

1. *Openness to surprises as opportunities for new ideas.* The leader must always be aware of the temptation to use existing or old mental models to look at new sets of circumstances. The leader's own mental model must also shift as the context tells a different story about experiences, reality, and the shift in emphasis or action.

2. *Situation testing in the validation of new information.* The leader is always testing assumptions, insights, and knowledge against a changing context. This contextual shift creates a demand to recognize that what one knows is not always constant. Information, data, and insights must be obtained as they arise and applied to the emerging situation so that there is a connection between context and action that is highly congruent and leads to good flow and appropriate action.

3. *Making accurate assumptions about new levels of uncertainty and inherent risk.* There are no risk-free actions. The leader must recognize that risk is embedded in every human activity and cannot be fully eliminated. Thus, the issue for the leader is a matter of degrees of risk rather than the elimination of risk altogether. Looking at levels and intensities of risk against required action gives the leader a sense of what will be required in terms of staff energy, commitment, understanding, and concerted personal action. This risk testing is a constant part of the leader's decision skills.

The leader looks for the relationship and integrity of linkage between all elements of work

Relational factors

Organizational realities

Personal realities

Synthesis of Organizational and personal realities

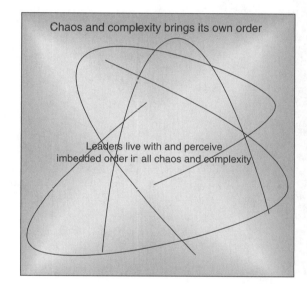

Chaos and complexity brings its own order

Leaders live with and perceive imbedded order in all chaos and complexity

Quantum Leadership Process

- Testing assumptions
- Reading signposts
- Stretching the limits
- Pushing perceptions
- Creating new mental models
- Reaching for the potential
- Behaving with boldness

Gem

Risk is embedded in every action. No change can occur at any level of the organization without a willingness to engage risk and maximize the benefit that lies secretly and deeply within.

4. *Evidence is in the action.* While the leader must consider all stages of decision making and consideration, ultimately, action is required. Most problems of leadership lie between the decision and action phases. Risk is embedded in all action taken. If no action is taken, then risk can be minimized or avoided, at least over the short term. However, there is a long-term price to be paid if action is delayed beyond the time of its demand. The leader looks at applying action at the right time. Timing is a critical strategy in facilitating and advancing vital change. Knowing when to act and how to act are as critical as is the action itself.

PATTERN RECOGNITION

Relying on outdated mental models and mind maps results in an orientation to the realities of the time. Entrenched thinking and outdated models are the result of not having kept up with changes in contextual issues and in patterns of work. Recognizing patterns is an important conceptual talent because it provides the leader an opportunity to understand what action is effective and when to take it. It helps keep the leader from undertaking polarized action or applying incomplete information to decisions. The leader that can recognize patterns in any given situation and synthesize the information those patterns demonstrate will make more accurate decisions. In this process the leader looks at the why of issues and sorts through the multiple arrays of information, determining what values and seminal elements can be drawn from it. The leader uses the aggregation of data and other complexes of information to create a mosaic, out of which can be drawn indicators of direction or supports for particular decision making.

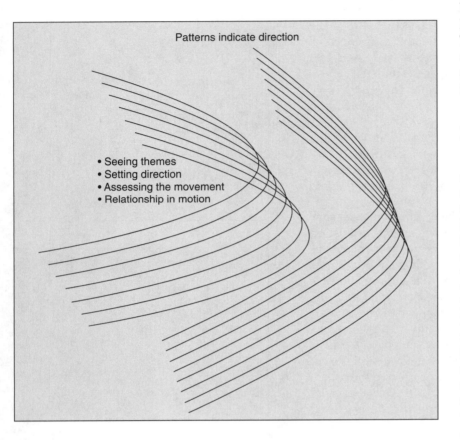

Patterns indicate direction

- Seeing themes
- Setting direction
- Assessing the movement
- Relationship in motion

SYNTHESIS

As leaders become more expert in systems thinking, they acquire the ability to synthesize many pieces of information into an integrated whole. Through analysis and integration, bits of information, pieces of data, elements of insight, and components of process can all be pulled together to help guide the imagination and thinking of the leader. Leaders take the various elements of information and draw relevance from them to guide their decision making and action. This synthesis of processes uses multiple sources as a way of drawing conclusions and taking action. The transforming leader applies systems thinking proficiently, moving past compartmentalization, incrementalism, and vertical models of thinking and planning to better delineate a goodness of fit between demand and action. Integration of thought and action are critical talents for the leader. Moving seamlessly through thought and application, the leader links as much data to current demand as possible so that action is always informed by the most vibrant and applicable supporting data possible.

Leadership Continuous Learning

1. Confronting the ritual and routine
2. Stimulating creative skills
3. Aggregating information resources
4. Applying all learning
5. Experimenting actions
6. Innovation thinking and application
7. No boundaries, lots of brainstorming
8. No permanent solutions or behavior
9. Using ambiguity to stretch assumption
10. Evaluating outcome and values

LEADERSHIP AND CONTINUOUS LEARNING

How often have managers confronted what appears to be "brain-dead people"? These are people who have become so addicted to ritual and routine they have no creative and responsive behaviors left to the demand for change. Here again the leader represents in the context of his or her own behavior a commitment to continuous adaptation and growth. In short, the leader indicates a personal availability to continuous learning.

Effective leaders continuously remain open to new ideas and approaches. In fact, they so live their availability to new ideas and approaches that it becomes their way of life. They represent to those they lead a living commitment to openness and learning. However, even leaders can experience information overload. With so much data unfolding at every moment of the workday, it can be hard to keep up with what the data is presenting. Often, the data itself becomes demanding, requiring time away from the usual activities of work just to be able to assimilate it and to organize it to make it useful. It is important to sort through desired information and useful information. The leader recognizes that there will be greater amounts of information available than individuals can use. It becomes the responsibility of the leader, therefore, to sort through the many sources of data and to discipline information flow so she or he can focus on those pieces of information that are important to particular moments or processes of decision making. This way, the leader prevents data backlogs and information overload. In the management of information, the leader uses time effectively by prioritizing the information that is critical to the work being done. Instead of simply reading journals, the leader pulls from the journal those articles that mean something in the context of the role or the demand of the time.

Data smog is an important issue for leaders. Not all data has value. Often data is generated to meet the needs of those sending it, rather than those receiving it. The recipient of data must make some decisions with regard to its value, meaning, and appropriateness to work demands. Leaders recognize information as a support service, not an end in itself. Careful management of what kind of information, what form the information takes, and what information has impact are basic requirements for making information usable. Leaders will find that most of the information generated has limited value. In fact, most of the information received will not contain anything of value at any given moment. Information, in fact, changes its value depending on the issues. It is the role of the leader to make sure that there is a goodness of fit between information used and the decisions made.

Leaders also need to sort in ways that help discern information that is real and that which is simply informative. It is wise to look at information from a questioning perspective, recognizing that information itself can be a source of problems. Information can be incomplete, inaccurate, or even biased. Leaders themselves can read information through biased eyes and therefore skew it in ways that reflect a particular perspective. There are critical differences between information management, developing knowledge, and obtaining a real understanding from appropriate utilization of data. Poor data and poor data management can get directly in the way of effectiveness and good decision making, especially if it crowds out good reflection, vertical thinking, appropriate dialogue, and openness to new learning.

Information tends to be seductive. Often, the more information one gets, the more seduced one is. What results can be an inability to recall or to recognize sources of information and to remember what information served as a basis for making specific decisions. There are several things

---

Openness to Learning

- availability to the new
- look past today
- moving past ritual
- questioning everything
- insatiable curiosity
- more questions than answers

Managing Data Smog

- sorting through the nonrelevant
- scrapping the unnecessary
- finding core information
- relating data elements
- using all the tools well
- don't accept the pieces till you've seen it all

Information Seduction

The appropriate management of information critical to the role of the leader. It is possible for information to the seductive and gamer data for decision-making that, if not carefully assessed, can lead to the decision maker in the wrong direction. The following elements are essential to avoid information seduction.

- check your biases
- makes sure it comes together
- read what the data actually says
- share it with others before acting
- reflect before acting
- listen to a different story from data
- draw different conclusions from expected

Information Leaders

- judicious review
- know what is right
- tie it together
- link the pieces
- apply data carefully
- make sure data is applied right
- data is reader/user friendly

Information Leaders' Problems

- being bombarded
- internal bias
- non-objective review
- make sure it's linked
- piecemeal presentation
- selective information
- incomplete data

Gem

Fear is like blinders over the eyes and the mind, binding you to past insights, practices, and experiences. Fear cripples the imagination and binds the spirit such that availability to the creative and the new is lost in the darkness of immobility.

a good leader does to compensate for the inappropriately dramatic impact of too much information:

1. *Discusses and compares information and data.* The good leader looks for opportunities to share information and insights, to obtain others' views, and to debate the veracity and impact of specific information on particular elements of work. This dialogue can offset dependence on e-mail, cell phones, message machines, and other mediums not requiring direct interaction.

2. *Makes time for personal reflection.* Understanding information calls for individuals to spend time with it to delineate its meaning. This level of meaning calls for a higher degree of reflection and discernment when one puts the information in the context of where and how it will be used.

3. *Looks to others to explain data that is difficult to understand or can only be comprehended through a different frame of reference.* Whenever there is information that is unclear, complex, or beyond easy understanding, the leader goes to those who can clarify and develop understanding in order to assure that the information always remains useful.

4. *Always asks how useful information is.* Getting information is not as important as having the right information and making use of it. As mentioned previously, sifting through information in order to find the riches that it provides requires that priorities be set with regard to meaningful information, avoiding seeking information that is not useful in the work or cannot be used for good decision making.

5. *Never allows her- or himself to be bombarded or held hostage to all the bits of information.* There is a level of insecurity that comes with not knowing everything. One of the obligations of social interaction is often being considered "with it" or "in the loop" regarding what's going on. The temptation to be drawn into this frame of reference is significant, especially considering the need for membership, inclusion, and social intercourse. Leaders, however, are constantly aware of the difference between that which is fashionable and that which is wise. The wise leader knows what needs to be known, relates that level of knowledge to the work and action that must be undertaken and the decisions that must be made. By keeping focused on this reality, the leader fails to be sucked into superficial knowing and fashionable response.

Fear is also a major impediment to openness and availability and to learning leadership. Fear usually generates from a few major sources. It is usually a response to an anticipated threat, discomfort, pain, or death. Fear can be so mobilizing that it can cripple appropriate decision making and action. Leaders recognize that fear is a constant companion in the human experience; it cannot be completely eliminated from our consciousness. However, fear can be either a motivator or an immobilizer.

Leaders should think about how they use their time and how their use of time reflects their confidence in how they deal with their own fear of taking action. Good leaders ask consistently: How do I do my job? What values about work and self were taught during my childhood? How was I dealt with in school? How did my peers perceive me and interact with me? Is my concept of self consistent with the demands on my role and my time? Am I skillful at prioritizing? Do I feel in control of my life and my time? How do I use my time to make sure that it is most effective? Self-reflection and the ability to think about values, meaning, and purpose have an impact on the legitimate expression of the leader's role.

Dealing with the personal anxieties of creating consonance between one's self-image and the expression of the leader's role is a critical process in advancing leadership effectiveness and obtaining leadership excellence. The leader who is not good at self-reflection is generally not good at leading others to make changes in their lives.

The strong leader makes self-reflection an active exercise and regularly schedules that as part of his or her leadership learning development. In this process the leader safely yet positively seeks information and support regarding skills, styles, and expression of the role. Good leaders accept the consequences of their own role and behavior, exhibiting a willingness to engage those consequences and to undertake action to compensate for whatever deficits or challenges must be addressed. Good leaders are familiar with the "no excuses" approach to learning. Nothing on the leader's agenda makes it difficult or increases the anxiety of confronting learning opportunities in a way that will produce meaningful personal and collective change.

PARTICIPATION COMPETENCE

In health care, professionals must be fully involved in the decisions that affect their practice and those they serve. Participation competencies require the fostering of good communication skills and the development of purposeful behaviors that promote professional commitment and action. Professional and personal goals must emerge so the level of congruence between the action of the professional and the goals of the organization can occur. High involvement is a requisite, not an option. People rarely become involved in those things that do not provide meaning for them. Restructuring organizations, changing the workplace, redefining work, or altering standards of work all have a direct impact on professionals attempting to do the work. Undertaking any of these actions without the concerted investment of those whom they impact is not a wise strategy for leaders.

High regard for engagement and inclusion is reflected in the role of the leader who emphasizes shared decision making and deliberate involvement of others in decisions. Embracing decisions independently is no longer an option in interdisciplinary and multifocal delivery systems. Large bodies of research exist that demonstrate that engaging and including professionals in making decisions improves the quality information processes, the application of good thinking, and the effectiveness of decisions and their implementation. The ability of the leader to view power within the context of the shared relationship is a vital notion to effective decision making in today's complex work systems. Work or involvement isn't an option for decision making; it is a mechanism for effective decision making that requires good skills and excellent process. The struggle is in moving out of parental behaviors and the leadership model that is based on hierarchical structures and parental frames of reference.

Leaders have to examine their own beliefs, as well as their attachment to certain behaviors and practices that may preclude equality and collaborative relationships in the workplace. Leaders must recognize that they are differentiated by role, not by position. Considering this, the leader recognizes that engagement in decisions that affect practice, work, or patient care must include those who are accountable for those activities. If high-quality outcomes are to be assured, those who do the work to achieve them must be fully invested in the decisions that affect them. Empowerment, accountability, and ownership are no longer additions to the excellent exercise of affective work. Leaders who are unable to incorporate such practices and behaviors into their own role simply can-

---

Self-Reflection

The strong leader recognizes that an important part of information management is reflection. This self-assessment should include personal biases, desires, and preferences. Looking past personal perspectives and reviewing the data within the context out of which it arises deepens the objectivity and clarity with which the leader can observe and assess the data. Critical components that should be carefully accommodated in this reflective self-assessment are:

- personal biases
- current mental models
- individual needs
- past practices
- self-fulfilling expectations
- wish listing
- prescriptive deliberation

Finding Meaning

We seek to find meaning in all we do:

- Look past the work and find the reason for doing it
- Seek the values embedded in action
- Reflect on the purposes related to doing the work
- Share insights with trusted others to give values a voice
- Challenge your beliefs regularly to validate them
- As leader, find others to explore new realities and insights
- Review values continuously

The Leader as Role

Leaders are simply playing a role they do not need to live every moment of their lives. However, every moment they are in the role they cannot pretend that they are not. Those they lead have a right to expect that they are leaders and will lead effectively.

Since it is a role, the leader may find time away when leadership is not expected in a place and time that is appropriate and away from work.

Interpersonal Competence

- Leadership is all about relationships
- Leadership requires emotional balance
- Conflict is present in all relationships
- Communication skills are not leadership optional
- The leader never owns others' issues nor resolves other people's problems
- Accountability means the leader sees that defined outcomes are attained
- Leaders have no friends; it is not a component of the role
- The leader keeps no secrets, in fact, favors disclosure

Facilitation Skills

1. Right people; right decisions
2. Good group-dynamic skills
3. Strong intuition regarding others' needs
4. Examine skill contribution of team
5. Mentoring and coordinating skills
6. Leaders favor no personal relationship
7. Leader models behaviors expected in others
8. Expected behaviors are defined in advance
9. Group goals are congruent with organization
10. Leader behaviors congruent with expectation

Quantum Leader Competence

- Technical proficiency in discipline
- Role understanding re: expectation
- Communication ability
- Discernment of direction
- Dialogue skill sets
- Coaching method and process
- Goal orientation
- Fiscal and goal congruence
- Systems facility and utility

---

not be successful in sustaining worker confidence and investment in advancing clinical care.

INTERPERSONAL COMPETENCE

Empowerment and participation cannot exist in practice if interpersonal facility is missing in the leader. In order to function well in the facilitating, coordinating, and integrating roles, a leader must be a masterful communicator. Interpersonal communication includes a wide array of relational and communication skills that result in constant investment and engagement and inclusion of individuals in decisions and actions that affect their work and their future.

Methods of communication and the framing of words and language are the major skills in communication and information management. Leaders are meaning makers and, thus, spend their lives translating strategies, decisions, and actions in the language of those who must live with the impact of the decisions of others. Reframing concepts and notions or reorienting language to express strategies and direction becomes a talent that the leader must develop to a high degree. This process of inclusion and relationship building is essential to the very ability of the organization to thrive. Negotiating, listening, setting others in internal compasses, reframing incorrect notions, reengaging others' principles, and translating strategy and direction into the language of practitioners are all basic skill sets of good leadership.

Facilitation and coaching skills require that the leader be able to form relationships with individuals and groups in which counseling, teaching, and mentoring is aimed at improving performance and more deeply investing the worker in the meaning and value of the work itself. Coaching and facilitating requires that the leader evaluate process rather than employee; sort through confidence, competence, and understanding to see that they are present in action; and identify and clearly enumerate performance problems as a way of developing insights into obstacles for good performance and developing tools for overcoming them.

LEADERSHIP COMPETENCE

There is no one set of activities or competencies that can fall under the rubric of leadership competence alone. Leadership competence is the sum of all the activities related to the expression of leadership covered in this chapter. Besides communication interaction, directing, discerning, dialoguing, and coaching the leader's ability to have a technical understanding of work and its application is clearly an important corollary to the expression of leadership. While it should not be the leader's expectation to be fully technically competent in all the elements of practice, or even of his or her discipline, it is important to be aware of the technical specifics that impact work. Staff have a tremendous appreciation for the exceptionally clinically skilled leader who not only expresses the role of the leader with great insight but can do it well within the context of the work expectations of clinical practice. This is a critical element of understanding what facilitates the positive impact of the leader's role.

Perhaps at the core of working with others are skills that relate to building and maintaining meaningful relationships and sustaining those relationships around the demands of work. Interdependence is a critical notion for successful leadership. Recognizing that all clinical activity is relationship dependent and fundamentally collaborative in nature, the leader ensures that such behaviors are consistently present. Leaders cannot avoid conflict (see Chapter 3). Relationship management and the intersections and interactions between individuals and disciplines is the critical centerpiece of all clinical activity. Leaders continually facilitate these intersections and broaden the frame of reference of those at the intersections. Bringing purpose, strategy, objectives, and a directional frame of reference to the work of staff helps connect staff to the broader journey of meeting the health care needs of the community. By doing this the leader maintains a meaning focus in the work of practitioners and makes that work congruent with the purposes of the health system.

Ultimately, from a systems perspective, the leader must continually integrate, facilitate, and coordinate between individuals and systems, seeking the highest level of convergence between making sure that the system supports the work of the individual and that the work of the individual fulfills the obligations of the system. All the support infrastructures, relationships, work processes, and clinical interactions must converge around the point of care in order to make sure that every effort interfaces in a way that meaningfully affects the delivery of patient care. It is there that good clinical leadership finds its fulfillment.

Leading from the Quantum Intersect

- integration of the disciplines
- group problem solving
- coordination of teams
- integration of service
- negotiating service boundaries
- mediating normative stressors
- generational integration
- goals achievement/evaluation
- facilitation of direction
- integrating conflicting demands
- continuous change management

A P P E N D I X 1

New Age Mythbusting

There are many who do not believe that the new age is here or that it is any different from any other time in history. In fact, there are those who would suggest that everything is simply a continuum of what has already occurred and that there is no real revolutionary elements that occur in the historical journey. Some even suggest that there is nothing new under the sun and that we have already experienced all there is to experience.

Of course, nothing could be further from the truth. The digital age has created a new level of reality, if not actually altered it forever. It is important for the leader to be able to perceive the drama of the changes confronting all of us and to engage its meaning and translate its application. But first, the leader must raise and confront the right questions about the myths and reticence before others are willing to engage the transformation in their own lives.

Myth 1: There is no change!

Leader questions:

What is it that is not changing?

How is your work different from what it was ten years, one year, three months ago?

How would you describe the world differently from your parents when they were your age?

What is different about work today from it was 100, 60, 30, 10 years ago?

Myth 2: Everything goes full circle and we end up doing it all over again, just like the last time!

Leader questions:

What exactly is it that we are doing that is the same as the last time?

Are the circumstances and conditions exactly the same as the last time, and will the response to them really be exactly the same?

How will we respond differently this time that will make the application of what we have already experienced unique to the time yet appropriate to the change?

Myth 3: I don't have to change!

Leader questions:

Can you remember what you looked like when you were 4 years old, 14, 24, 34, etc.? Do you look the same now?

Have you watched your children age, grow, change, become adults? Are you exempt from that same process?

Work always changes; how do you change with it to continue to be relevant or valuable?

Myth 4: I dream of the good old days!

Leader questions:

Which one?

Are you willing to live with what wasn't available to you in the good old days?

Can you accept the bad as well as the good of the "good old days"?

Is it possible for you to visualize what things were really like in the good old days and place yourself in the midst of them? Describe everything those days represent.

Myth 5: Our quality of life is in decline!

Leader questions:

How is your life less than what is was 50, 30, 10 years ago?

Name the conveniences you have now that you didn't have 30, 20, 10 years ago.

Name at least two medical treatments available today that weren't available 10 years ago.

What would you be willing to give up in your life that allows you to live better and more comfortably, if you went back 30, 40, 50 years ago?

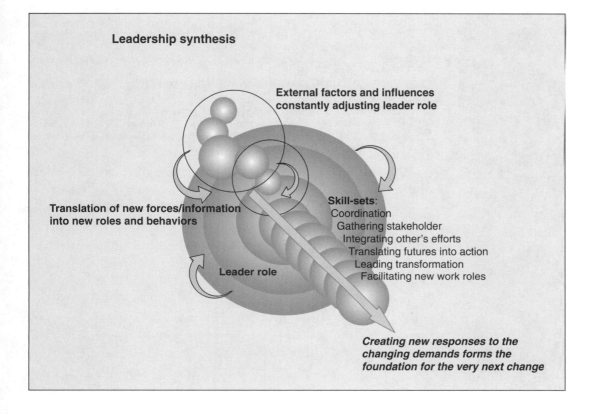

Leadership synthesis

External factors and influences constantly adjusting leader role

Translation of new forces/information into new roles and behaviors

Leader role

Skill-sets:
Coordination
Gathering stakeholder
Integrating other's efforts
Translating futures into action
Leading transformation
Facilitating new work roles

Creating new responses to the changing demands forms the foundation for the very next change

SUGGESTED READINGS

1. Avolio, B. J., & Yammarino, F. J. (2002). *Transformational and charismatic leadership: The road ahead* (Monographs in leadership and management). Boston, MA: JAI Press.

2. Bryner, A., & Markova, D. (1996). *An unused intelligence: Physical thinking for 21st-century leadership.* Berkeley, CA: Conari Press.

3. Laub, J. A. (1999). *Assessing the servant organization: Development of the servant organizational leadership assessment (SOLA) instrument.*

4. Thompson, C. M. (2000). *The congruent life: Following the inward path to fulfilling work and inspired leadership.* San Francisco: Jossey-Bass.

5. Henry, C. R. (1996). *A general reflects on leadership and management: Reorganizing, consolidating, downsizing.* Columbus, OH: Battelle Press.

6. Austin, D. M. (2002). *Human services management: Organizational leadership in social work practice.* New York: Columbia University Press.

7. Bhal, K. T., & Ansari, M. A. (2000). *Managing dyadic interactions in organizational leadership.* Thousand Oaks, CA: Sage Publications.

8. Zaccaro, S. J., & Klimoski, R. J. (2001). *The nature of organizational leadership: Understanding the performance imperatives confronting today's leaders.* San Francisco: Jossey-Bass.

9. Sagini, M. M. (2001). *Organizational behavior: The challenges of the new millennium.* Lanham, MD: University Press of America.

10. Porter, L. W., Angle, H. L., & Allen, R. W. (2003). *Organizational influence processes.* Armonk, NY: M. E. Sharpe.

11. Fairholm, G. W. (1993). *Organizational power politics: Tactics in organizational leadership.* Westport, CT: Praeger.

12. Murensky, C. L. (2002). *The relationships between emotional intelligence, personality, critical thinking ability and organizational leadership performance at upper levels of management.*

13. Romig, D. A. (2001). *Side by side leadership: Achieving outstanding results together.* Austin, TX: Bard Press.

Quantum Leadership: Effective Conflict

CHAPTER OBJECTIVES:

Upon completion of this chapter, the reader will:

1. Define the elements of conflict and the applications of each element to the work of leadership.

2. Outline the elements of response the leader must make to adequately address the components of conflict.

3. Develop the leadership role in normative conflict management by developing conflict processes as a tool for effectively managing differences.

4. Construct a program or approach to normative human conflict that is ongoing and operates as a fundamental part of conducting the business of providing health care.

INTRODUCTION

In making conflict normative, the leader creates a frame for conflict that turns it from an event to a process. The more conflict is looked at as a normal occurrence, one that reflects the usual vagaries of human interaction, the more likely it can be handled appropriately.

CREATING A CONFLICT-FRIENDLY CULTURE

The good leader recognizes that conflict cannot be avoided. In fact, this leader does everything not to avoid conflict. What the leader does is create an environment that provides a safe space for identifying and expressing conflicts. This leader recognizes that conflict management is the one fundamental obligation that he or she has in the leadership role. Knowing that conflict cannot be avoided, the leader makes it comfortable and safe to engage conflict at any stage. More importantly, this leader recognizes that opening the staff to the noise, ambiguity, and challenge of expressing differences creates a special milieu, which, in turn, can often be demanding for the leader to manage.

> The best way to avoid conflict is to create a culture where conflict is accepted as a part of the way of interacting with each other.

Addressing Potential for Conflict

In this stage, leaders are required to:

- Develop their intuition and use conflict resolving processes
- Keep an eye on what's going on
- Listen to staff clues of conflict
- Note the differences that are causing "noise"
- Remember always that the leader does not own the conflict
- Create an atmosphere of trust
- Remember that diversity is essential to all good dialogue
- Ensure that communication is open and honest

Intuitive Potential for Conflict

- *Awareness* of individual needs
- *Sensing* shifts in communication levels
- *Notation* of personality differences
- *Noticing* clique formation
- *Seeing* whispered conversations
- *Hearing* sarcastic comments
- *Observing* change in relationships
- *Watching* increased negativism
- *Detecting* decrease in satisfaction

Isolating Conflict

looking for the potential:

- Anticipating differences
- Change in language
- Change in feelings
- New processes
- New employee
- Shifting priorities
- Critical event(s)
- Personality clashes
- New work demands
- Loss(es)

Good leaders are responsible for creating a positive context for work. Leaders are continually attempting to provide a framework for work that is positive, encouraging, and growth oriented. A good part of creating this context is building the kinds of relationships that evidence partnership, openness, and trust.

When conflict is considered a regular part of the manager's responsibilities, confronting it directly becomes a part of expressing the manager's role. The manager must begin to recognize that fear of confrontation is a significant impediment to resolving interpersonal and relationship-based conflicts.

The best time to address conflict is early in its expression. Seeing a conflict situation emerge, is a forewarning that it is likely to blossom. The manager needs to know that conflict does not go away of its own volition. Since it is normal for almost all human interactions, conflict simply changes its form and emerges somewhere else or in some other kind of "wolf's clothing."

The longer conflict simmers, the more difficult it is to resolve. Conflict is not a static process that just sits there, failing to gather energy. On the contrary, it is not uncommon to watch unresolved conflict grow in intensity as it lies just below the surface collecting energy and building toward a cataclysmic eruption. Unresolved conflict always intensifies.

The good leader has an intuitive sense of the potential for conflict. This person knows that every interaction is rife with the seeds for conflict. Human differences drive its unfolding. If not recognized early, the conflict continues to gather potential and to grow in possibility until its expression becomes likely. The leader wants to do two things in the presence of the potential for conflict: address it early and address it appropriately.

SKILLS FOR ISOLATING CONFLICT

Leaders need to recognize that early engagement of conflict means recognizing it soon enough to address it without "noise" and/or overwhelming personal emotion. In the earliest moments of an interpersonal conflict, the beginning signs of the impending conflict are always present. If an attitude of disrespect is evidenced, an unkind word from one person to another is said, an offhand remark uttered, or an inappropriate phrase communicated, all of these and more can be early signs of the gathering storm of a conflict. The leader lets no remark or behavior that represents anger, misunderstanding, or personal apprehension go unaddressed. Each of these emotions is an indicator of an underlying set of concerns that begs to be addressed. Interrupting the course of a conflict in these early stages gets the real issues out in the open and raises the chance that addressing them will allay further opportunity for the conflict to accelerate.

From constant awareness to listening carefully to the content of the conflict, the leader prepares to mediate the conflict in the right manner. It is important for the leader to be able to identify the key elements of the impending conflict situation. What most often appears in the conflict is usually the signpost that the real issues lie somewhere more deeply buried. The leader may need to dig further to find the critical source for the conflict. Usually conflict language represents feelings, not circumstances. Feelings generally either get in the way of the truth or actually mask it.

The leader may need to go through the feelings in order to get to the underlying issues in order to really resolve conflict situations. There are trigger remarks that are indicative of intensity of feeling and perception that the leader will need to sort through. Often the leader will first hear feeling responses:

"She always does this to me."
"He is forever dumping on me."
"She never stops criticizing me."
"He makes me so angry."
"She makes me just want to scream."
"He swears at me all the time."

These comments are filled with reactive emotion. They represent feelings of anger and even helplessness. Sometimes they are accompanied by behaviors; sometimes they are merely expressive of feeling. Either way, they are powerful indicators of impending and irresolvable conflict.

Not all conflict can be addressed by the leader on the spot. Work requirements may mean that the conflict expression temporarily goes in the "parking lot" of response until it can be more reasonably addressed. Even so, if the leader hears the comments from the aggressor or from the offended individual, it is important that a response be identified regarding follow-up action. Short yet key responses to the individual(s) from the leader are advisable.

To the aggressor:

"I'm concerned about what I just heard; I'll need to talk with you about it after we finish this task (work, procedure, meeting, etc.)"

Or

"I hear what you're saying and I think we need to talk about it after we are done here."

Or

"I am very unclear about what you are saying here and I think we need to talk about it right after we're done here."

The leader might respond to the offended person:

"I need to know more; let's talk when we're done here."

Or

"I'm concerned about how you're feeling right now. Let's talk when this task (meeting, procedure, work, etc.) is finished."

You'll note that the leader does not yet address the two (or more) individuals quite yet. There needs to be more clarity built around the conflict before any purposeful resolution occurs. Getting the facts and feelings straight from the outset will be a critical element in the resolution process. Perhaps the most important aspect of getting conflict straight is found in correctly gathering the right information. The good leader pays attention not only to what is said but also to what is felt. Getting to what is said is always best obtained by going through the individual's feelings first, so that those feelings have a route of expression, clear content, and the individual has an opportunity to be heard early in the process. Too often, leaders try to resolve the conflict early on, hoping that by doing so they can shortcircuit the conflict and keep it from escalating. As a result, leaders often fail to address strongly felt personal feelings that, if left unaddressed, ultimately affect the sustainability of conflict resolution.

CREATING A TRUSTING CONTEXT

Building a great conflict resolution process is the one thing that assures conflict is minimized. In health care, focusing on the patient requires a strong trusting relationship between and among all staff members. Staff members who work in an atmosphere of distrust do not collaborate or integrate with each other in providing care and reaching organizational goals. In the presence of rapid change, a level of distrust and uncertainty can quickly and easily emerge.

The willingness and ability the leader can gather to assure staff commitment, energy, and mutuality clearly affects the quality of staff mem-

Always keep an eye out for these emotional trigger words—they are telling the leader that conflict is emerging and feelings are growing more intense!

Gem

The leader is aware that conflict is always present regardless of the lack of evidence of its action. Anticipating the action of conflict is central to the role of good leadership. The leader never forgets the continuous and inevitable role of conflict in all human interaction.

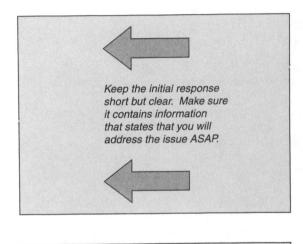

Keep the initial response short but clear. Make sure it contains information that states that you will address the issue ASAP.

Gem

Unresolved conflict always gathers energy and continues to grow in intensity. Always!

Gem

Do not resolve conflict too early in the process. If you fail to manage all the essential steps, the conflict will strike back later in a way, a time, and a place you never expected.

bers' work. There are specific behaviors that break trust between people and can create a milieu rife with conflict.

Unfair Procedures and Processes

Any time staff perceives that work rules are unfair or inappropriately applied, elements of mistrust emerge. In these circumstances, staff began to feel that their opportunity in providing input and making a contribution to the work is limited. This begins to interfere with their ability to communicate and interact confidently with each other. When the leader has her or his own agenda or undertakes individual action processes out of context with the rules of the organization, elements of mistrust emerge. Consistency, fairness, equal application of the rules, and open communication help maintain an environment of trust that encourages the staff to ask questions, approach the undiscussables, and explore difficult issues together.

Not Communicating Fully

When all staff members can openly communicate and share information interactively, they create a spirit of inquiry and open information sharing. In this way, all members have an opportunity to obtain and make use of all the information necessary to work well and to achieve meaningful outcomes. These behaviors actually facilitate trust and build a foundation for expanding trust between and among team members.

The leader must always be alert to the cues that indicate that openness in relationship and communication is not operating effectively between and among staff members. Some signs are:

1. silent response to a statement or question
2. nodding with no actual verbal acknowledgment
3. labeling staff members as "non-team players"
4. language games and jargon
5. staff members disappearing in the presence of other staff members or the leader

These behavioral indicators tell the leader that trust is lacking between and among staff members and that further addressing of the environment of communication is required to adequately maintain effective communication and interaction.

Allowing Alienation between Individuals

Relationships between and among staff members are important to their ability to work together effectively over the long term. Any problem or struggle in the relationship eventually breaks down the whole team's ability to communicate and work together. The leader wants to address any issues of discomfort, relationship problems, and ineffective communication as quickly as possible. As with all conflict, issues will grow into major problems fairly quickly. Emotional challenges that exist between individuals also reduce each person's opportunity to develop the trust they will need to effectively undertake their work.

Misguided Focus of Staff

Staff members have their own assumptions about what should be accomplished and how the work should be done. With professional staff,

---

The Price of Distrust:

- Untenable noise
- Lack of involvement
- Crisis in confidence
- Noncommunication
- Personal isolation
- Errors in practice
- No team consciousness
- No loyalty
- Limited accountability

Addressing Interpersonal Alienation

- Make sure expectations regarding communications are precise and clear
- Include communication effectiveness as a part of the competency-based performance requirements
- Make all staff accountable for communication and interaction problems between any staff members
- Keep the team focused on its contributions and the individuals value to the team
- Do not let personal behaviors, agendas, and values impedes staff members ability to interact and communicate effectively
- Address isolation and alienation behaviors immediately

the notion of individual intent and professional self-direction often predominates. This may cause the individual staff to undertake action independently or individually in a way that is not appropriate or in the best interests of the organization and those it serves.

The leader must recognize this issue early in the staff behavior pattern. Unilateral and individual performance expectations or actions that are not in concert with standards or team expectations can create great interpersonal noise in the organization. The leader must be able to clearly recognize the individual professional staff member's need for self-direction and decision making, yet provide a context within which those decisions can be deemed appropriate and valid. Addressing these issues in advance of performance by using clear protocols, policies, and practices helps provide clear and effective parameters for individuals, which helps identify the boundaries of performance and individual behavior.

Eliminating Superior-Subordinating Behaviors

Health care is rife with historical hierarchical structures, roles, and relationships. These traditional practices have unfolded over a long period of time in health care and have created conditions and circumstances that result in "master-servant" relationships, behaviors, and patterns of interaction. Because control is such an integral element of hierarchical relationships, certain individuals reflect a higher level of need for control and controlling behaviors. Other staff members are more passive and are therefore more easily managed and controlled by others. In either case, the behaviors are inappropriate in any effective professional environment. Quantum leadership is about building relationships and intersections and establishing the patterns of communication and response that reflect the nature of these relationships.

It is important for the leader to ensure that these behaviors are not represented in her or his own leadership. The leader must be careful to remove maternalism/paternalism within the leader's own specific pattern of behavior. The leader must clearly articulate in personal behavior a pattern of partnership, collegiality, and professionalism. Through representing this pattern of behavior, this leader creates a milieu and a set of expectations with regard to the partnering behaviors asked of the staff. Eliminating old hierarchical behaviors is extremely challenging in an environment that has historically valued and embraced them. For the leader, it will always be a work in progress, exemplified by her or his own personal behavior and relationship with the staff.

Eliminating Word Games

Language is critical to the effectiveness of organizations. It is the means within which understanding is obtained, communication is advanced, and action is taken. Precision and clarity in the expression of language, especially in a professional environment, is essential to maintaining the value of the work. Often, however, in the work environment, language and words are not as deeply valued as they need to be. The careless use of language can lead to misunderstanding, errors, and missed opportunities for accomplishment.

Sometimes, purposeful distortions and misuse of the language can be undertaken by staff, and even leaders, ultimately distorting meaning. Using doublespeak as a means of deliberately clouding the message; jargon to indicate a unique or special use of the language; or complex, refined, and manipulative use of words can operate in an individual's best interests and significantly affect others' understanding and action.

Addressing Staff Misguided Focus

1. Watch individual practice making sure it is consistent with standards
2. Listen to other staffs, and complaints about an individual's performance
3. Make sure protocols, policies, and practices are clear
4. Identified limits and boundaries to practice or work
5. Assure a model for mentoring and precepting is available to new staff
6. Identify models and mentors for practice and relationship behavior
7. Support staff who question and challenge practices and protocols and explore options to questionable practices and processes

---

Eliminating Superior/Subordinate Relationships

- Reduce or eliminate as much hierarchy as possible
- Emphasize partnership in communication and decision making
- Clarify expectations with regard to professional behavior
- Reduce and ultimately eliminate parentalism and leader behaviors
- Help staff develop increasing collateral interdependence in both decisions and professional actions

---

Managing Word Games

- Make effective communication a clear expectation of team relationships
- Create a continuing dialogue around clear and effective communication
- Directly and immediately confront individuals who frequently use language as a weapon or personal tool
- Help staff develop techniques of validation clear and effective communication
- Clarifying meaning in all questionable communication or information that is ambiguous or unclear

---

Gem

Either locating or laying blame has absolutely no value in the action of problem solving. Undertaking blame-based processes always guarantees that staff will avoid confronting legitimate issues and problems with an attitude open to obtaining meaningful solutions and sustainable problem resolution.

Effective Listening Tips

- Keep focused on the facts
- Look for both the meaning and the feeling of the words you're hearing
- Inhibit your desire to immediately respond
- Clarify quickly when you don't understand
- Don't allow eyes to wander; stay focused on the subject
- Lean into the conversation; body language is important
- Make no judgments, just listen
- Take notes if you find it helpful

Quantum Tips

Like most things in life, timing is important when effective listening is required. Make sure that important messages are not delivered in the midst of chaos or intense business. Find a place that is quiet enough to enable concentration and conversation.

Language games are the most frequent tools used by those who have need for control or wish to express their own personal agendas at the expense of the relationship with their colleagues in the organization. The leader must address these activities as soon as they appear so that their legitimacy never gets initially established.

Eliminating Blame

The presence of blame is always an indicator of the lack of accountability and the clarity necessary for responsibility to be ascertained and appropriately expressed. Blame is always a sign of ineffective valuing of contributions and roles in the organization. Furthermore, it is an indicator of the lack of accountability embedded in the organization's values. Locating blame rarely leads to or sustains effective problem-solving process. In the presence of blame, individuals flee from problem identification, solution seeking, and corrective action. The good leader recognizes there is no value in blame and works diligently to remove blame strategies from the organization's patterns of working behavior. Here again, the leader eliminates blame-based activities and responses as quickly as he or she sees them.

THE VALUE OF EFFECTIVE LISTENING

Listening is a fundamental and essential tool of good leadership and conflict management. The listening demeanor, which essentially encapsulates the leadership role in active listening, is one of the most effective leadership devices to incorporate as a conflict skill set. However, listening is frequently more difficult than most leaders realize.

Rather than a passive function, listening is actually an active process. It is a discipline. Listening requires a level of openness and awareness that is critical to effective communication. Most people treat listening as a passive exercise, more receptive than active. Effective listening is reflected in the ability to take in the full expression of communication that comes from another individual, recognizing that listening has a visual as well as aural capacity. The active listener is constantly screening the full expression of communication. Looking at gestures, body language, verbal cues, and intensity and method of expression is all part of effective listening. Managing conflict is, perhaps, more precisely specified in this facility for effective and active listening.

Often the single greatest problem with regard to listening is also its simplest: Most people simply don't want to listen. Talking is often perceived as a much better experience than listening. However, the good listener plays a much more powerful role in the management of information and the circumstances of communication.

The leader should be listening at least 50% of the active time in a leadership role. While this is a minimum, it does give the leader an opportunity to evaluate the degree of listening that she or he brings to the role. There are some measures that can help with delineating awareness related to the leader's level of listening effectiveness:

- *Note your interruption quotient.* Frequent interruptions are an indicator that effective listening is not occurring. Usually high-level interrupters are more interested in what they have to say than to what they have to hear. Assessing and measuring the interruption level or intensity in the individual leader's self-expression can be a clear indicator of listening effectiveness.

- *Ask others about your own listening skills.* The good leader will ask someone he or she trusts about specific personal listening skills. It is important that the leader be specific when asking about listening skills. It might even be wise for the leader to ask a friend to call or watch the leader listen and to make evaluative comments related to the style of leader's listening and suggest improvements or changes that could occur in the personal listening style.
- *Develop self-awareness regarding your listening process.* Periodically the leader should undertake a self-assessment regarding the listening approach. Self-monitoring body language, level of understanding, awareness of the other person's style of communication, and the ability to effectively condense and articulate what is being heard are all tools to help the leader assess listening skills. In this process, it is often helpful for the leader to ask the person communicating for information about her or his own assessment of the leader's presence, awareness, and responses to the individual's effectiveness of communication.

There are a number of listening mechanisms that, when left unexamined, create some real problems in assuring communication effectiveness. The leader must examine these challenges to communication in her or his own behavior and also the behavior of staff. Effective listening communication behaviors are simply the first line of defense in managing conflict effectively. The following should be red flags:

- Clearly not wanting to hear what someone is sharing and actively defending oneself against what one is hearing. This mechanism can impede the availability of and willingness to listen effectively.
- The method of communicating that one is listening to may be personally irritating or uncomfortable. This generates a desire to be nonresponsive and not present to the message or the messenger.
- Feelings of being overwhelmed and tired can make the listener not available to the message. Increased levels of response or energy may not be readily available in a particular moment of communication.
- Anticipating one's own answers while listening to the message is a great impediment to effective communication and listening. Getting ready to give an answer before listening completely is one of the most frequent barriers to effective listening.
- Past practice, or past habits of listening that have been unaddressed for a long period of time (past listening rituals) can be one of the great barriers to developing healthier, more effective mechanisms for listening.
- Preconceived notions about what is being heard or about the person communicating can limit availability to hearing what is really being said. Judgments made about the person can impede the value of his or her message.
- Diminishing the value of the messenger can often limit how one listens and how much one hears. Devaluing the communicator always diminishes the value of that person's message.

Conflict resolution is embedded in the ability to really hear and understand the messages that underlie any element of conflict. In order to respond well, the manager dealing with conflict must be able to hear and understand a multitude of messages that indicate the underlying issues or concerns between and among people. Being available to others, open to their needs, positioned carefully to hear what it is they have to

---

Barriers to Effective Listening

- External stimuli like sound, light, voters, mannerisms, inflections, and movement
- Mind sets, the listeners emotional and mental characteristics and responses
- Language clarity, ambiguity, misinterpretation contributing to level of understanding
- Feedback elements such as premature responses or comments, early listener evaluation, feeling responses (resentment, defensiveness, suspicion, etc.)

Good Listening

1. Stop talking—listen
2. Put the communicator at ease
3. Make sure you want to hear the message
4. Limit distractions
5. Focus on the other person
6. Patiently hear
7. Assess your emotions
8. No judgment
9. Ask questions for clarity
10. Count to three before you respond

Listening

Donna is trying to let Marie know that she is going to need some help in understanding her patient's diagnosis. She has been attempting to explain her understanding to Donna at the nurses' desk. While Donna is taking, Marie has been doing her charting, answering a call bell, sending off a lab request, and checking a medication request. Marie has been shaking her head as Donna speaks, but keeps on with her activities.

How do you feel about Marie's listening posture?

Is Donna's message likely getting through to Marie?

What is a better approach Donna's and Marie's interaction?

Conflict and Listening

- Seek to clearly understand
- Clarify for a real meaning
- Look for the deeper message
- Always listen between the lines
- Listen from your heart as well as your head
- Distinguish between facts and feelings
- Empathize, not sympathize
- Make sure your listening is goal directed
- Remember conflict involves more than one person, listen to all messages

Note-taking in Active Listening

- Assess intensity or emotions in situation
- Keep notes short and point-based
- Reflect back to individual what you have written
- Review notes taken between parties to validate critical points

Cycle of Positive Conflict Process

1. Underlying issues in person or values
2. Differences emerge between persons
3. Differences are manifested in behavior
4. Conflict emerges and escalates
5. Conflict affects relationships or processes
6. Need to address conflict arises
7. Mediation of conflict
8. Solutions are explored
9. New directions or patterns are established
10. Evaluation indicates change effectiveness and indication of next steps or further actions

say, and clear that the messages heard are important considerations in effective conflict management.

Body language and perceptive availability are critical elements and signs of readiness to listen. Paying attention to whether arms are crossed or relaxed; whether posture is slouched or the listener is sitting straight ahead and leaning into the conversation, facing the speaker directly and closely; and whether the listener is making continuous and focused eye contact are all indicators to the communicator as to whether the listener is fully available and listening to the message.

Some leaders who are active listeners always carry a small notebook in their pocket for such purposes. These people recognize that not everything that is said can be heard and remembered over time. While the context of the conversation and the needs of the communicator must be taken into consideration when taking notes, note-taking is a valid way of exemplifying your presence and your willingness to hear. Simply because note-taking does not occur frequently enough reduces others' perceptions and expectations that it is either permissible or viable. The leader makes it clear and safe for listener and communicator to use whatever mechanisms better assure that communication has been properly heard and noted.

It is appropriate for the listener to consciously and infrequently ask questions to clarify the content of the message. The infrequency and precision of questions is a clear indicator of whether the mechanism is successful in expanding and validating what is being communicated. It also serves as an exemplar with regard to the level of intensity of listening and of clarifying what is being heard. Rather then open-ended questions, the leader should be precise and specific, using questioning as a way of clarifying and understanding the specifics of the message. As always, questioning joins with awareness, presence, focus, availability, body language, and openness as the foundation and framework for effective listening. Without having refined the tool of effective listening to a high degree, the ability to undertake meaningful conflict resolution is measurably limited.

IDENTIFYING THE CYCLE OF CONFLICT

Like any other human dynamic, conflict has content, particular elements, and specific processes. Kinds of conflict generally fall into relationship-based, value-based, structural-based, data-based, and interest-based categories. Each one has its own characteristics and elements that mark it as unique. The leader becomes skilled at identifying the kinds and characteristics of conflict being dealt with and the responses that best address them.

Since the leader is always looking for specific conflicts, it is wise to become skilled in identifying the particular characteristics of conflict that most often appear within the culture of the service or department. Each setting is unique with regard to the makeup of the staff and the stressors on them and the work that they do. The good leader makes a "conflict potential" assessment as a part of delineating which strategies are going to be most helpful in dealing with conflict. In this assessment, the leader is attempting to get a handle on those specific potentials for conflict that will most often be a concern in the ordinary management of the service.

The leader looks at the makeup of the staff, the demographics (both cultural and age-related), the breadth of the work, and the skill level of the staff. Embedded within these factors is the potential for specific kinds of conflict that may recur. In this manner, the leader makes the potential for conflict a normal and usual part of her or his organizational and resource planning. This leader knows that the greater the awareness of the circumstances and characteristics of conflict, the earlier it can be addressed appropriately.

Relationship-based Conflicts

In any work environment, there are a number of personalities and situations whose vagaries create conditions that can lead to conflict. Differences between people always provide a source for a variety of relationship-driven crises or conflicts. Differences in personality create problems in interaction and communication and often lead to misunderstandings. These differences can frequently lead to specific altercations reflecting emotional involvement and personal animosity. Left unaddressed, these differences can escalate and create real polarization between the involved parties and those who relate to them. Relationship conflict is the most frequently experienced conflict in most organizations. Communication irregularities emerge and miscommunication becomes common. Negative behavior becomes repetitive and, if not resolved, becomes a way to sabotage and offend the opposing party, which can affect the work, workers, and those they serve.

The good leader recognizes the potential for this conflict early in the process. Usually unkind words, snide comments, asides, negative comments to others, and avoiding behaviors are the early signs that a relational conflict is present. Since the leader always expects some level of conflict to exist, she or he is able to see these signs and begin to take action right away.

The leader will first want to get at the originating source for the conflict. Confronting both parties separately with regard to the behaviors expressed is the critical path to getting at the root problem underlying the behaviors. Beginning the questioning with an open-ended approach is best:

I'm noticing that . . .
Can you tell me . . .
I'm wondering if I'm seeing . . .
Help me if I'm perceiving this right . . .

At this stage, the leader is just trying to get a level of understanding about the existence of a problem and the basic perceptions of what the problem might be through the words of each party. Through this process, the leader is simply validating whether a problem exists and the underlying nature of the concern. The leader is also ascertaining the degree of perceptive agreement that exists between the parties regarding their issues.

The leader initially responds to emotions and feelings. It is impossible to get at the problem without first going through the emotional content of each party's issues. In relationship conflict, the parties are reacting to their own feelings and impressions of what has happened to them and how they are feeling about it, rather than to the real issue that may be the causative factor. If the leader tries to get to the causative issues too soon, the parties may block and refuse to move there since they have not had an appropriate opportunity to work through the emotional content related to the issue.

Sometimes the leader might need to carefully move individuals through their feelings by validating and supporting the person while clarifying the underlying issues along the way. The leader attempts to get the individual to a more reality-oriented place from which some rational work might be done as they move through the conflict. At some point, the parties must be in the same place in order to move the conflict closer to resolution. The leader attempts to prepare each to understand where both individuals are in relation to feelings and content. The leader, acting as a

---

Assessing for Conflict

- Define cultural and age demographics of staff
- Determine level of work intensity
- Look at range of staff skills
- Review staff longevity
- Assess amount and rate of changes occurring in the service or department

---

Look for Early Signs of Conflict

Potential for conflict

Look for:

- Negative behavior
- Secret conversations
- Exclusion from groups
- Whispering
- Open fighting
- Snide comments
- Sarcasm
- Strong language
- Changed body language

Look for How People Are Expressing Emotions and Feelings

Important Emotions

Look for:

- Passive feelings
- Crying
- Anger
- Fear
- Threats
- Silence
- Sarcasm
- Physical tension
- Running away

Rules of Engagement

- Open dialogue
- "I" statements only
- Ownership of own feelings
- Openness to differences
- Hearing the other
- Must remain present
- Truthfulness
- Equity in relationships

Creating a Culture of Acceptance

- Evidence of fairness
- Ownership of feelings
- A level "playing field"
- No favoritism
- Balanced exchange of views
- Safe place for expressing feelings
- Good conflict processes
- Focus on solution seeking

neutral, will seek to have each party express his or her feelings with a language that accurately expresses feelings without further polarization, energizing a new level of emotional intensity.

As the process moves toward engagement, the leader seeks to focus on expression and "rules of engagement" as well as to remind each party of the expectations regarding communication and conflict management in the service or the department. Having created an appropriate milieu for conflict management, the leader wants to ensure that the parties are aware of the expectations and of the need to resolve issues that impede the ability of the staff to communicate and deal with differences. The leader identifies the conflict resolution process as one of the mechanisms that exemplify the components of communication within which the unit operates. It is only at this point that the leader begins to bring the parties together to dialogue and work through their differences.

Values-based Conflicts

Perhaps one of the most difficult classes of conflict to resolve is one that represents differences in values. Every person brings different experiences and beliefs to the expression of their human journey. Cultural, social, religious, moral, and personal values are all part of what defines an individual. In a multicultural society such as that reflected in the American experience, cultural and personal differences are a common experience. Yet with the richness of these differences comes the inevitable conflicts that arise when individual values come in conflict with the values of others.

The leader creates a culture of acceptance and openness to differences and to the vagaries of response they reflect. In anticipation of the potential for conflict, the leader sees to it that cultural and value awareness is inculcated into the educational and developmental activities of the service. Everyone should be expected to participate in activities that teach them about the value and practice of acceptance and about the behaviors that are forbidden between and among different ethnic, cultural, national and religious groups.

Because value-based conflict is so difficult to resolve late in the cycle of conflict management, it is wise to confront it at the earliest possible moment. A breach in the code of conduct or expectations of behavior should be addressed as soon as it happens. The absolute unacceptability of such patterns of behavior should be clear to everyone at the outset. Refusal to conform one's personal behavior to these rules of good relationship should be grounds for the strongest disciplinary action.

Ethnic irregularities have no room for dialogue or debate. Any discrimination based on color or disparaging remarks that reflect on ethnic origins have no room for misunderstanding. In a world of many colors and ethnic backgrounds reflecting the broadest array of human beings, any conflict based on this has no room for negotiation and misunderstanding. In the human experience, there are some "a priori" considerations that operate beyond question. Race is one of them. The only room for conflict in this arena is where a misunderstanding or misrepresentation of one's remarks or behavior has occurred and needs clarification and restating between the parties. Cultural or language difficulties or misrepresentations can create a perception that simply may not have been intended. The process of continuous cultural and values education for staff should keep such misunderstanding to a minimum.

Religious and values differences can create significant problems. There are a number of problems that can come out of religious differences related to beliefs, practices, and accommodation. Special considerations to religious and values practices can create negative feelings in others who do not hold the same beliefs. Resentments and feelings of preference can emerge, creating conflict. Here again, being clear in advance about what the expectations are regarding the presence of staff with different practices and the impact of those on the staff relationship is a critical obligation of the leader. Adjustments required in the schedule, and even assignments and role adjustments, need to be clear to all staff members with attention paid to how equity is maintained between and among staff members. Achieving equity between and among staff members with different religious or values needs is challenging for the leader and the staff. Dialogue and negotiation regarding these adjustments must be delineated up-front with the staff. This approach keeps the issue before the staff, makes it a part of their ongoing work experience, and creates an expectation that such accommodations are always a part of the work environment.

When accommodations to the expression of particular religious practices is especially difficult or verges on creating resentment, the leader must reanimate dialogue around the differences in light of reinvigorating acceptance and undertaking creative ways of addressing the related issues and resolving the conflicts these issue generate. If the leader has been successful in the aggressive creation of an environment of acceptance and openness, the expectation is that such problems can be dealt with and ultimately resolved.

In cases where there is intractable religious-based conflict, it is often wise for the leader to expand the dialogue and include experts from outside the service to guide the discussion and advance resolution. It is often helpful to involve pastoral assistance from representatives from the religious traditions at issue and have them help the participants find some common ground and define areas of resolution or accommodation. The leader always acts as a resource purveyor when resolution processes require an alternative mechanism for resolution.

In values-based conflicts, it is also helpful for the leader to expand the dialogue to values that can be shared by all participants. Those values that operate in the broader human context and reflect common human needs and interests can help refocus the issue to one that engages human experience, regardless of value tradition or expression. Attempting to find common areas of value (such as family, home, nation, loyalty, sentiment, children, etc.) can change the emotional and relational content of the conflict and create a common frame of reference for its resolution that might not have been originally anticipated.

Finally, it is important for the leader to know that it is sometimes necessary to allow people to agree to disagree. Values are sacred to the individual who holds them; they can't easily be surrendered to others. The leader may have to get the parties to determine how they will live with their differences and make the necessary accommodations to those differences as a part of their relationship. Respect is critical to effectiveness of this process. If each can respect the position of the other, common ground can be found and progress can be made with regard to the quality of the work relationship.

Structure-driven Conflicts

These conflicts recognize inequities inherent in the system or structure of work. These can be classified as inadequate or unfair policies, processes, rules, behaviors, and practices, as well as contextual and organizational factors that inhibit cooperative relationships.

Scenario

Marie, the nurse manager, is working to create an atmosphere for resolving conflict between two of her staff members. She is getting the room ready for the mediation dialogue. Marie will facilitate the mediation, she is busy thinking about the process and how to make it favorable for dialogue and solution-seeking. She is a little tense about the process but realizes that her recent certification in workplace mediation will be helpful in facilitating this process. She has made the room comfortable with chairs facing each other and with herself placed in the middle seat to guide the interaction. Marie has thought about each step of the process and reminded herself not to take a position and to stay focused on managing the dialogue and keeping faithful to the steps by step process of dialogue and movement to resolution.

Key elements for Marie to address:
- comfort of participants
- peacefulness of the space
- use of the conflict process
- keeping the discussion focused on the issues
- help explore alternatives to original positions
- allow feelings to be expressed
- support participants as they move through the process
- clarify issues, enumerate progress
- define solution, expectations and follow-up on actions.

Dealing with Religious Values and Language in Conflict Situation:

1. Set the language boundaries
2. Don't allow one participant to hold others hostage to particular beliefs
3. Focus on issues, not beliefs
4. Stay centered on tangible issues
5. Keep dialogue directed to how issue will be resolved

Dealing with Values-Based Conflicts

1. Look at the why and the who issues
2. Discuss tangible solutions that can be seen clearly by all parties
3. Find common issues and values
4. Link common values where they can be found
5. Keep dialogue centered on "core" causes and drivers

Gem

Everyone shares some common value with others. The good mediator is always looking for something that ties the parties' experiences together so it can help anchor further dialogue and assist in identifying common ground.

Confronting Imbalances

- Eliminate favoritism
- Balance dialogue
- Remove status barriers
- Find a common language
- Keep issue centered
- Limit unrelated dialogue
- Call parties by first or last names
- Remove any status symbols
- Reword for increased understanding

Hidden Conflict

- Favoritism
- "Class" levels of employeeism
- Status barriers
- Differentiated benefits
- Professional cliques
- Management secrets
- Management control
- Exclusionary behaviors
- Extreme executive perks

Structural Conflict

- Inadequate architectural design
- Bad policy requisites
- Inadequate procedures
- No guidance for action
- Bad management practices
- Poor support services
- Inadequate communication
- No electronic clinical record
- Poor problem-solving processes

The leader recognizes that no workplace is free of structural and operational challenges to the ability to do work and to build relationships in the system. Differences in pay grades, benefits policies, reward systems, job and role status all contribute to perceptions of structural inequity. Even if there is a rational basis for these practices, the inherent inequity needs to be addressed as a possible source of unresolved conflict.

The leader recognizes that there must be openness with regard to people's specific concerns regarding any particular structural inequity. The leader acknowledges its presence and clearly enumerates the logic behind the apparent inequity. Understanding the value of implementing a particular advantage by one group in relationship to others is a valuable first step. In those places where the inequity established is sufficiently egregious, mechanisms and efforts at self-correction must address the structural element. Where such inequities can be changed or struck down in the organization, they should be, as soon as possible, with a solution that can be implemented.

There is a perceived inequity and imbalance at the professional level of a number of organizations. These perceived imbalances generally indicate that one profession or work group is preferred or treated favorably compared with another profession or work group. This perceived inequity often creates much internal conflict in the organization that may not always be directly expressed. Its hidden conflict operates as an organizational subtext or frequently lies just below the surface. In this specific set of circumstances, the leader must recognize the foundations of the perceived inequity early and clearly. If it is status inequity evidenced by differentiation and role or reward, the justifications and support for these differentiations must be clear enough to make sense to the group that feels disadvantaged. While these inequities cannot always be changed or altered, they can be understood. The role of the leader is to generate such understanding.

Where there are more challenges in justifying the inequity and it does not appear to be legitimate or functional, the leader must support individuals in undertaking a process in which the inequity can be actively addressed and pursued further. In such circumstances, advocacy for a particular approach or solution, communication with the appropriate leadership individuals, or structural or organizational approaches to finding solutions must be determined by the stakeholders in the conflict. Without the leader advocating for a specific process for problem resolution, the structural problem will continue to frustrate and challenge the effectiveness and integrity of the work group

Additional structural challenges that can generate conflict relate to the environmental or the architectural construct within which work unfolds. In many clinical organizations, the structures of the organizations themselves impede the effectiveness of the work. Where the structures can be altered, they should be. Where the architectural and structural elements of work cannot be altered or adjusted, mechanisms and methods for accommodation or modification must be explored by those affected by the structural impediments. In addition, continuing leadership attention and focus must be centered on addressing the structural barrier in a way that ultimately removes it. This emphasis indicates that the leader is committed to supporting the clinical work. The leader also represents in this activity an understanding that these issues are part of her or his role in continuously challenging those structural elements that do not support the clinical work of the organization. Whether the architectural modifications or structural adjustments can be undertaken is not as important as the commitment of the leader to continuous support of the staff by challenging organizational leadership to modify structural impediments as evidence of leadership's commitment to the clinical work of the organization.

Interest-based Conflicts

Conflicts that reflect an interest foundation are generally caused by a mutual commitment, yet conflicting relationship, to a shared interest. In health care, each interest-based conflict can take on the mantle of professional boundaries and turf protection. Each practice profession attempts to advance its interests in undertaking the work of patient care. In so doing, the boundaries between the professions become clouded or at least uncertain. As these boundaries become less firm, the potential for conflict begins to emerge. Because all the professions are interested in advancing their own role in rendering effective patient care, their interests can frequently conflict. Adding to this significant concern is a long history of hierarchical relationships between and among the disciplines in a very structured health delivery system. Such controls were originally designed to protect the interests of physicians in undertaking their clinical work. Physicians historically have operated at the apex of the clinical hierarchy, based on the assumption that by virtue of education and role they are clearly most advantaged in managing and controlling the clinical activities of the patient. However, over the years, as care has broadened and become more complex, the hierarchical model and unilateral locus of control by the physician is no longer adequate in meeting the needs of the patient. More interactive-based approaches to delineating and delivering patient care are now requisites for practice. Having failed to resolve boundary conflicts at earlier levels of the relationship, contemporary conflicts accelerate in intensity and passion as the issues become critical to the practice roles of the individual professions. Professional capacity, competence, and ability to perform the work are now limited by the various professions' availability to each other and the lack of technologies and methodologies for resolving these role-based interest conflicts.

The leader has a special set of challenges in bringing together disparate groups in an effort to resolve boundary and relational issues between them. However, this work must be considered as fundamental to the role of the leader in every clinical setting. Furthermore, the leader must help the professional groups supply time and commitment to addressing the specifics of the conflict that may impede their ability to relate and impact patient care. The leader must have the groups focused on their common interests, such as advancing patient care efficiency or effectiveness, rather than allow them to continue to focus on their positions. This creates some common ground upon which solution can be sought. In addition, the leader must help the groups deal with their resolution by using objective data. This translates passion and feeling derived from an experiential or perceived framework into a framework reflecting data-driven evidence regarding actual activity and its impact. Building a data-generating process (research) helps create the objective framework around which differing groups or professions can converge. In health care, the generation and use of objective data can provide a strong framework for common action in the resolution of interest-based conflicts.

In interest-based conflict management, the leader focuses on solutions that address the broad needs of all the parties, based around their common interests such as patient care. Calling the stakeholders back to those issues and keeping them focused on their mutual impact can help the leader in moving the parties to common resolution. In undertaking this approach, the leader will need to recognize that the offering and management of trade-offs, options, and alternatives will be a necessary part of the conflict interaction between groups that express differing or conflicting professional interests. While keeping the groups broad-based and focused on impact and outcome, each will reflect on what will have to be sacrificed or traded in order to find common ground. Groups keep score,

---

Resolving Interest Conflict

- Identify interests
- Have parties own their issues
- Give feelings ample play
- Clarify role in the conflict
- Find common themes
- Use the parties language
- Identify critical event(s)
- Anticipate personality clashes
- Enumerate new work demands
- Give time to express loss(es)

Working with Disparate Groups

- Name their "frame of reference"
- Identify needed "gets" early
- Balance "feeling" issues
- Name the boundary issues
- Enumerate common themes
- Find common language
- Look for conflict "triggers"
- Reduce personality clashes
- List expectations of each party of themselves and of others

---

Interdisciplinary Conflict Considerations

Each discipline has its own content and contextual boundaries that define it. The leader recognizes the real value members have for their intra-disciplinary identify and relationships. Members will bring these parameters to the conflict table and will hold onto these identifies. The leader looks for the "boundary" issues early so that dialogue around interfacing at the boundary and reestablishing new intersections or roles there can be discussed and resolved. This is especially true as practice changes are challenging what professionals do and is changing their interactions and relationships almost daily. The leader will need to be especially adept at anticipating these conflicts and get to them as early (before, if possible) as possible. Late engagement of these conflicts can result in high "noise," extended conflict and challenging resolution.

and the leader should too. Any inequity in the number and kinds or significance of trade-offs will be noted by the parties and will dramatically affect the ability of the leader to move them to common ground and conflict resolution.

The leader must always recognize that these conflicts are dynamic; that is, they are continuous, and one level of resolution always leads to a higher level of dialogue and more intensive conflicts. As the complexity of care and service becomes more intensive, so do the conflicts associated with them. The leader, therefore, establishes an ongoing mechanism or format for continuous dialogue and interface between the involved disciplines as a mechanism for assuring that the normative conflicts of multidisciplinary practice are addressed as an ordinary and usual part of doing the business of the clinical organization.

Data-based conflicts

Conflicts related to data are generally driven by either limited access to information or lack of information. Information is critical to the effectiveness of organizations in today's clinical workplace. Without appropriate information in a useful configuration, clinical work cannot be successfully undertaken. In fact, the complex of information necessary to do the work now makes the work completely information dependent. This information is critical to the ability of any of the disciplines to fulfill their obligations in rendering clinical service throughout the health-care system. Furthermore, business, clinical, support, and material information must interface in order to create a sufficient data foundation upon which effective clinical choices can be made. It is this generation and interface of information that creates some of the most difficult and intractable problems and conflicts.

Information is resource intensive. As a result, there are wide variabilities related to the distribution and quality of hardware and software across the health-care system. Emphasis has historically been placed on building a business infrastructure and information system, and much business sophistication has emerged as a result. Clinical information infrastructures are just now being expanded and linked to business infrastructure in ways that can have an impact on resource use and clinical decision making. However, information priorities, mechanisms for generating information, distribution of resources in building information infrastructures, and the quality and kind of information generated all have an impact on organizational effectiveness and integrity. Therein lies the source for the emergence of conflict. Each of these issues can generate its own internally fixed sources of conflict from access, availability, accuracy, quality, efficacy, and utility of information.

The leader must recognize that a fit is necessary between resource allocation and information usefulness. Since there are intersecting groups, all requiring various components of the information complex, some level of agreement must be achieved as to what information is necessary, important, and vital to clinical decision making. Agreements between organization-established priorities and clinically useful data processes and information must be interfaced in a way that is resource wise and reflects service utility. In addition, the leader must ensure that there are structural and process formats, within which these priorities and elements should reflect the useful and common set of criteria to which all stakeholders have contributed. The leader's role is to reduce the structural opportunities for conflict by assuring that appropriate processes and interfacing regarding information collection, management, and generation have been effectively delineated and structured within the organization. The leader makes sure

---

Continuous Dialogue

1. Regular meetings wit staff
2. Make differences OK
3. Create safe space for dialogue
4. Mix the disciplines in dialogue
5. Use flip chart to record process
6. Use effective/proven processes
7. Have staff lead discussions
8. Set priorities for problem solving
9. Meet with dialogue leaders before formal meeting with others
10. Always make conflict normative

Gem Useful Information

The great conflict leader is always aware of the power of effective information. No conflict dialogue should progress without the most accurate information necessary to validate process and progress. Information is the most powerful tool in the conflict process. The leader seeks it, gathers it, presents it at the right time, clarifies it when it is ambiguous or seeks more of it when it is inadequate. Resolution is a truth-seeking process. There is nothing more devastating that resolving a conflict on a false premise—for process must always begin again. The opportunity to recover the energy of the first resolution is difficult, if not impossible to regain.

that the right stakeholders are at the appropriate table so that deliberations include those upon whom decisions will impact. When issues have been overlooked or forgotten, the leader, recognizing the process is fluid, brings the stakeholders together again to deliberate and reassess with the intent of establishing a process which works successfully. Where there are challengers to the skill set and ability of the stakeholders, the leader assures that appropriate experts and expertise is available in order to guide the team to correctly delineate needs and resolutions with regard to information management solutions. Through this complex of activities and systems approaches to handling the information infrastructure, the leader creates an ongoing mechanism that embeds conflict resolution in the information system utilization process.

In each of these arenas are specific and unique activities related to resolving the conflict. While this workbook certainly introduces some of the steps that can be undertaken by leaders to address conflict, it isn't a comprehensive reflection. The leader must recognize that conflict management is a significant skill set and obtain as much development and education as necessary to build conflict management skills. Facility in conflict management comes with discipline, practice, and time. The leader, recognizing how important conflict management is to successful group interchange and group dynamics, therefore commits considerable time and energy to understanding and developing those skills.

The Leader Creates Sustainable Solutions

The leader is committed to creating an environment where solution seeking is the normative pattern of work behavior. The leader seeks to maintain a healthy environment for the conflict process to be integrated into the business practices of every service or department. When all is said and done, an ongoing dynamic of development and skill building in conflict processes is a normal part of the function and learning activities of the organization. At a minimum, the leader assures that the following should always occur:

- Staff remains skilled in conflict identification
- Managers maintain expectations and processes for conflict resolution
- The department remains a safe place for addressing differences
- Actions are followed up
- Continuing education includes conflict skill development
- Shared decision making works
- Role/performance expectations are continuously negotiated
- Manager-staff interaction occurs frequently.

Information-Systems Value in Conflict

1. Creates opportunity for access
2. Links and integrates information
3. Is a vehicle for common problem responses
4. Is data rich
5. A common tool, useful to all participants
6. Can make data conflicts clearer
7. Supporting source for objective information
8. Immediate implementation of many solutions
9. Reduces ambiguity of inputs or responses
10. Useful for evaluation of outcomes/ effectiveness

Gem

Leaders engage and embrace conflict as a regular component or the array of leadership tasks. Building the dynamic or conflict resolution into the practices of the department or unit creates the milieu for staff that makes conflict "safe" and expects that it will be dealt with as a regular part of the function and operation of "doing business."

REFERENCES

Kossgard, M., Schweiger, D., & Sappienze, H. (1995). Building commitment, attachment, and trust in strategic decision-making teams: The role of procedural justice. *Academy of Management Journal* 38(1), 60–85.

Moore. C. (1996). *The Mediation Process: Practical strategies for resolving conflict.* San Francisco: Jossey-Bass.

SUGGESTED READING

Kossgard, M., Schweiger, D., & Sappienze, H. (1995). Building commitment, attachment, and trust in strategic decision-making teams: The role of procedural justice. *Academy of Management Journal* 38(1), 60–85.

Marcus, L., Dorn, B., Kritek, P., Miller, V., and Wyatt, J. (1995). *Renegotiating healthcare: Resolving conflict to build collaboration.* San Francisco: Jossey-Bass.

Moore. C. (1996). *The mediation process: Practical strategies for resolving conflict.* San Francisco: Jossey-Bass.

Rothman, J. (1997). *Resolving identity-based conflicts in nations, organizations and communities.* San Francisco: Jossey-Bass.

Weisbord, M. (1992). *Discovering common ground.* San Francisco: Berrett-Koehler.

CONFLICT SCENARIO-ORGANIZATIONAL CONFLICT

Sam had been on the critical care unit for 3 years and had just received his advanced certification in cardiac critical care. He was excited by the opportunity to move to the Cardiac Care Center after reading a personnel posting of a new position for an advanced cardiac nurse within the Cardiac Care Center. Sam immediately submitted his credentials and his application for the position. He was interviewed by the nursing staff from the Cardiac Care Center and by their management team. At the completion of the interview by the management team, Sam was assured that the position was his and that he could count on hearing from them shortly about his having obtained the position.

Two weeks passed and Sam still had not heard any news with regard to his application. He called the human resource department and was informed by them that someone else had been selected for the position. Sam was hurt and upset by the news. He informed the human resource officer that he'd been assured after his interview with the nursing management team that the position was his. Since that time he had merely been waiting to hear confirmation as to when he might begin his new position in the Cardiac Care Center. The human resource officer assured Sam that unless he'd received formal confirmation from the human resource office he could not anticipate that the promise of a position have been made. This news caused Sam to be further upset and concerned with regard to the potential for this new position.

The more Sam thought about this the angrier he became. His hopes had been high, he'd obviously interviewed well and been well received, and yet still did not obtain the position. Furthermore, he felt that he had been promised the position based on his interview performance. What made him even angrier was that no one bothered to communicate either positively or negatively with regard to his application for the position before it had been offered to someone else. Upset with this set of circumstances and concerned about his future, Sam petitioned for a formal mediation in an effort to resolve his conflicting concerns.

Scenario Exploration

Clearly there are a number of issues involved in Sam's experience that raised the potential for conflict. Spend some time discussing the issues and circumstances related to this scenario and the places where the potential for conflicts is embedded.

1. What was the first moment that indicated a potential for conflict?
2. What was missing in the interview process that facilitated the potential for conflict?
3. What actions in the interview process helped create subsequent conflict?
4. What did Sam do/not do to participate in creating the conditions for conflict?
5. What are the critical elements resolving this conflict?

Undertake a role-play process in relationship to this conflict. There should be three members of the role play. (Sam, human resource department representative, and mediator), and each role should be rotated among the members of your group. Initiate a formal conflict resolution process using the principles identified in this chapter. Follow the process template contained at the end of the chapter. Discuss both the process and the outcome of the mediator role play.

CONFLICT SCENARIO-RELATIONSHIP CONFLICT

Fran's story:

Fran had been an exceptionally competent charge nurse on the neuro unit for 10 years. She had never had any problems with new staff. There had been plenty of them over the years, many coming and orienting to the nurse role fresh out of school and, after a year or two, leaving as quickly as they had come. Fran did not lament the movement but saw it as a normal part of developing a nursing career. She saw herself as a mentor for these new nurses and was hopeful that her role modeling was well received and that those she coached operated at a skill higher level after their experience with her.

Debbie was a different case. Since she had shown up, she created nothing but stress for Fran and the rest of the staff on the unit. Debbie had a chip on her shoulder the size of a redwood and took no counsel from any of the staff. She acted as though she were better than everyone and could do no wrong. Every time Fran approached Debbie to advise her of some issue of practice or new opportunity for learning, Debbie appeared distracted and acted as though she wanted to run. Debbie would speak out during clinical rounds declaring everything she knew about the diagnosis or care needs of the patient being discussed. She constantly interrupted and corrected other staff when she thought they were wrong. Whenever Fran tried to talk about Debbie's behavior, Debbie would tell her to mind her own business and suggested that she might want to attend to her own practice instead of critiquing others' work "all the time." Fran thought this woman had better get a different attitude or she wasn't long for this place. One more "crack" from Debbie and Fran was going to blow up at her. And not a moment too soon from Fran's perspective.

Debbie's story:

This was Debbie's first role as a registered nurse in primary care. She had graduated at the top of her class and had always been under the gun to perform well and to be the best nurse she could be. Her mother always insisted that Debbie be the best and do the best in everything she attempted. And Debbie had been the best from the first grade all the way through college. She has to continue that effort in this new job, especially when so many counted on her doing the best clinical work she could muster. This first job was her foundation year in the profession and it was very important for her to prove herself.

If only Fran would leave her alone. She was always looking over Debbie's shoulder snooping around for trouble. Fran always seemed to find out what Debbie was doing wrong and seemed happy to point it out to her. Even when Debbie contributed to the clinical rounds, Fran would have something negative to say. What did Fran know that Debbie didn't know, anyway? Debbie wished Fran would stop spying on her and simply leave her alone. Fran was just trouble and kept wanting to make trouble for Debbie. What was she going to do about her?

Scenario Exploration

Take a look at this scenario and discuss its implications from the perspectives of both Fran and Debbie. As a group, explore the following questions:

Describe how each person sees themselves in the their roles.

How does each person view the other's role? Is it accurate? In what way do they differ?

continues

CONFLICT SCENARIO-RELATIONSHIP CONFLICT
continued

What are the errors each has in the perception of the other?

How do the misperceptions drive the behavior each has toward the other?

What are the real underlying issues affecting their relationship?

How might you suggest the mediation process to each of these nurses?

Break up in groups and take turns doing a role-play mediation of this scenario. Evaluate each other as you follow the mediation process and apply it to this case. Please note: there is no right answer to this case, just one that works for the participants. Share your perspectives on the case and the mediation process at the completion of the exercise.just one that works for the participants. Share your perspectives on the case and the mediation process at the completion of the exercise.

Workbook Conflict Template 1

The Conflict Resolution Cycle

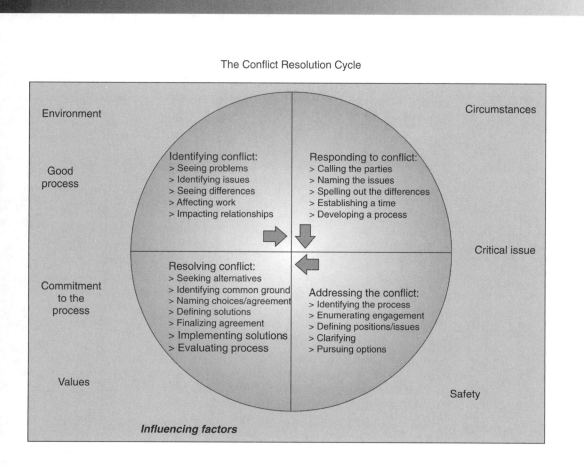

Environment

Circumstances

Good
process

Identifying conflict:
> Seeing problems
> Identifying issues
> Seeing differences
> Affecting work
> Impacting relationships

Responding to conflict:
> Calling the parties
> Naming the issues
> Spelling out the differences
> Establishing a time
> Developing a process

Critical issue

Commitment
to the
process

Resolving conflict:
> Seeking alternatives
> Identifying common ground
> Naming choices/agreement
> Defining solutions
> Finalizing agreement
> Implementing solutions
> Evaluating process

Addressing the conflict:
> Identifying the process
> Enumerating engagement
> Defining positions/issues
> Clarifying
> Pursuing options

Values

Safety

Influencing factors

Workbook Conflict Template 2 Follow a Process for Conflict Resolution

Eight Steps to Conflict Resolution

1. Make a safe space for conflict resolution process
   - Comfortable
   - Quiet
   - Caring
   - Open
   - Prepared
2. Get a basic understanding of issues
   - Issues
   - Feelings
   - Elements and details
   - Reality base and clarity
3. Name individual needs
   - Needs identified in parties' own words
   - Needs parties have of each other
   - Perceptions of meeting needs
   - Clear up misperceptions
4. Identify expectations from each other
   - Name the "gets" each wants
   - Sort through the differences
   - Identify resource issues
5. Clarify alternatives
   - Identify critical issues
   - Name the alternatives
   - List the remaining issues
   - Check off the differences
6. Bridge
   - Finding common themes/ground
   - Hidden "gems" of agreement
   - Affirmations of common interests
7. Define agreements
   - Generation of alternatives
   - Selection of alternatives
   - Determination of priorities for action
8. Finalize agreement to action
   - Finalizing agreements

- Determining parties' actions
- Acting on agreement
- Evaluating process
- Follow-up on agreement actions

SUGGESTED READINGS

1. Deutsch, M., & Coleman, P. T. (2000). *The handbook of conflict resolution: Theory and practice.* San Francisco: Jossey-Bass.
2. Diehl, P. F., & Lepgold, J. (2003). *Regional conflict management.* Lanham, MA: Rowman & Littlefield.
3. Drafke, M., & Kossen, S. (2002). *The human side of organizations.* Upper Saddle River, NJ: Prentice Hall.
4. Fenn, P., & Gameson, R. (1992). *Construction conflict management and resolution.* New York: E & FN Spon.
5. Fredrick, C., & Atkinson, C. (1997). *Women, ethics and the workplace.* Westport, CT: Praeger.
6. Fujishin, R. (2001). *Creating effective groups: The art of small group communication.* San Francisco: Acada Books.
7. Gorden, M. (1972). *Comparative political systems: Managing conflict.* New York: Macmillan.
8. Green, R. L. (2001). *Practicing the art of leadership: A problem-based approach to implementing the ISLLC standards.* Upper Saddle River, NJ: Merrill.
9. Gudykunst, W. B. (1978). *Bridging differences: Effective intergroup communication* (3rd ed.). Thousand Oaks, CA: Sage Publications.
10. Hare, A. P. (1992). *Groups, teams, and social interaction: Theories and applications.* New York: Praeger.
11. Honeycutt, J. M. (2003). *Imagined interactions: Daydreaming about communication. Interpersonal communication.* Cresskill, NJ: Hampton Press.
12. Jones, T. E. (1999). *If it's broken, you can fix it: Overcoming dysfunction in the workplace.* New York: Amacom.
13. Kalbfleisch, P. J., & Cody, M. J. (1995). *Gender, power, and communication in human relationships.* Hillsdale, NJ: Erlbaum.
14. Kellett, P. M., & Dalton, D. G. (2001). *Managing conflict in a negotiated world: A narrative approach to achieving dialogue and change.* Thousand Oaks, CA: Sage Publications.
15. Levi, D. (2001). *Group dynamics for teams.* Thousand Oaks, CA: Sage Publications.
16. Linstead, S., Fulop, L., & Lilley, S. (2004). *Management and organization: A critical text.* New York: Palgrave Macmillan.
17. Rahim, M. A. (2001). *Managing conflict in organizations* (3rd ed.). Westport, CT: Quorum Books.
18. Richman, L. (2002). *Project management step-by-step.* New York: Amacom.
19. Stewart, J. R. (2002). *Bridges not walls: A book about interpersonal communication* (8th ed.). Boston: McGraw-Hill.
20. Watkins, M., & Rosegrant, S. (2001). *Breakthrough international negotiation: How great negotiators transformed the world's toughest post-Cold War conflicts.* San Francisco: Jossey-Bass.

The Vulnerable Leader

CHAPTER OBJECTIVES:

Upon completion of this chapter, the reader will:

1. Develop an understanding of the value of leadership vulnerability as it relates to current health-care organizations.

2. Apply skills in becoming more vulnerable and open to risk taking, using focused leadership scenarios.

3. Learn new techniques of information management, overcoming silence, assuring an ethical climate, and recognizing cosmology episodes to mediate leader risk.

4. Reinforce the value of the characteristics of high reliability organizations as essential quantum leader tools.

INTRODUCTION

I don't have all the answers; am I a failure? Traditional organizations hold leaders to standards of rationality, clarity, and foresight—yet most leaders cannot meet these standards because they are human and face an incredible amount of unpredictability and fallible analyses of data. To be able to prosper and thrive in the millennium, the leader must shift from the somewhat comfortable position of control to one of great uncertainty and vulnerability. In reality, uncertainty and need for vulnerability has always existed for leaders. With the current explosion of information technology and availability of information, the choice to lead using command and control behaviors is no longer an option. To be sure, no leader is alone in this journey. Colleagues, patients, and the community are aware of the plethora of data, data sources, and lack of clear pathways.

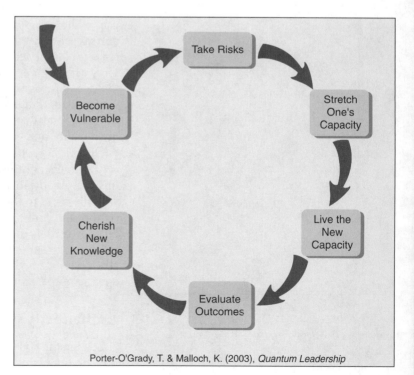

Porter-O'Grady, T. & Malloch, K. (2003), *Quantum Leadership*

A New Lens for Leaders

Openness to new ideas requires skills embedded in the acceptance of vulnerability and all of the emerging realities that are encompassed in the cycle of vulnerability (Porter-O'Grady & Malloch, 2003). Yet, most leaders believe that others expect them to have answers, to know the needs of the future, and, of course, to make money! When faced with the reality of the uncertain marketplace, most consumers are seeking honest and authentic leaders, not clairvoyants or charismatic magicians. Consumers recognize the uncertainty and, given the probable impact on their personal future, want to be a part of making decisions that impact their health. Consumers do not want to be mere recipients of healthcare plans created for them without their input.

The phases of the vulnerability cycle are presented as distinct entities for the purposes of discussion only. In reality, they are more often seamlessly linked. The six phases in the cycle are: becoming vulnerable, taking risks, stretching one's capacity, living the reality, evaluating the outcomes, and cherishing the new reality. Then the cycle begins again. The vulnerability cycle offers a new lens through which leaders can examine and evaluate leadership behaviors of both themselves and members of their team. Each phase will again recur with new situations and new strategies for the quantum leader to thrive on (Porter-O'Grady & Malloch, 2003).

VULNERABILITY

Vulnerability and Bad Leadership

While traditional leadership views vulnerability as a weakness, the new age of leadership embraces vulnerability as an essential competency. The notion of the vulnerable leader does not equate with bad leadership. The vulnerable leader of the quantum age is open to all realities, is collaborative, and aware of limitations. In contrast, the *bad leader*, or bad leadership, is characterized by the power wielding of Richard Nixon; the master communications manipulation of Hitler; the tyranny of Howell Raines of the *New York Times*; those who do not address known dishonesty of their employees; or Kozlowski of Tyco, whose impudence, greed, and tax evasion resulted in criminal indictments (Kellerman, 2004). These leaders could have benefited from a greater understanding of vulnerability as a key leadership trait, evidenced by openness to others, to new ideas, and recognition of limitations. Vulnerability is a more appropriate way to lead, rather than through manipulation to protect one's reputation, dishonest communication to deceive others, arrogance, believed invincibility, and outright greed.

Of great importance is the reality that leadership is not a moral concept; leaders are trustworthy and deceitful, brave and cowardly, generous and greedy. To assume that all good leaders are good people is to be willfully blind to the reality of the human condition and also limits our opportunity for becoming more effective at leadership (Kellerman, 2004). Further, leaders must remember that just because they are leaders, they are not necessarily trustworthy, brave, and generous and never deceitful, cowardly, or greedy. The recognition of fallibility allows leaders to manage the human condition and ultimately achieve greatness.

Authenticity is the Key

Leadership styles, among them autocracy, democracy, and situational, provide templates for behavior. None, however, are absolute or appro-

---

Vulnerability

Traditional Characteristics

- Weakness
- Open to or defenseless against criticism
- Susceptible to being wounded or hurt physically
- Susceptible to temptation or corrupt influence

Quantum Characteristics

- Openness to others
- Openness to new ideas
- Aware of limitations

GEM

If they can't trust you, why would they ever follow you?

priate for all situations. This plethora of leader styles can be daunting for the emerging leader. Formal monitoring programs provide guidance and recommendations to support role development. Yet, conforming to the normative leadership style of the organization or the recent literature recommendation can spell disaster for the leader. According to George (2004), great world leaders all had very different leadership styles—George Washington, Winston Churchill, Margaret Thatcher, Mother Teresa, and John F. Kennedy all led in their own unique way.

In reality, the success of the leader is more closely linked to personal authenticity than it is to a particular leadership style. It is your authenticity, not your leadership style that really matters. Attempting to emulate another's leadership style can be disastrous. New leaders may desire a model of shared leadership but must understand and live the basic values in their personal lives in order to make shared leadership a reality. A lack of congruence between personal and professional values creates a reality gap that is obvious to team members. This gap compromises leader authenticity, as the leader talks the talk of shared leadership but is unable to fully live the values consistently.

The values of the authentic leader are shaped by personal beliefs and developed through study, reflection, and dialogue with others. These values create a moral compass for the leader and provide guidance in determining the right thing to do rather than blindly attempting to emulate the style of another leader.

A broad understanding of leadership styles serves merely as background information to understanding behavior options. Being your own person is the key to developing an authentic leadership style that is consistent with your personality and character. Ongoing development of one's personal leadership style continues as different situations and different people are encountered.

The authentic leader accepts personal faults as well as strengths and avoids attempting to win approval of others by covering up shortcomings and thus sacrificing authenticity to gain respect from others. There is no way a leader can do everything, be on top of the incoming mail, read the most recent literature, and be responsive to everything and everyone; attempting to be such a leader is only fooling yourself. The authentic, vulnerable leader knows what he or she knows, what he or she does not know, and is content with the limits of his or her capacity.

Integrity is closely linked to authenticity for the effective leader. In addition to personal authenticity, the vulnerable leader emulates integrity, a characteristic that is not just the absence of lying but the presence of telling the whole truth, no matter how difficult it might be. Leadership integrity is the uncompromising adherence to moral and ethical principles. From authenticity and integrity, trusting relationships emerge.

The next section of this chapter presents specific leader vulnerability behaviors that will further enhance vulnerability as a very positive characteristic.

LEADER BEHAVIORS

Vulnerability: Mindfulness for the Right Signs

Every signpost or red flag in health care does not require attention and action. One unhappy patient or disgruntled employee should be noted; whole systems analyses should not be undertaken when other processes are working well. For example, if one visitor of ten thousand complains about parking proximity, a full-scale analysis of parking conditions is not needed. The complaint is data to be considered and then be aware of for

---

Quantum Gem

Information voids will be filled by rumors and speculation unless they are preempted by open, credible and trustworthy communication. Pull no punches. When you know an answer, give it. When you don't, say no. When you're guessing, admit it. But don't stop communication.

Jean B. Keffeler

Dimensions of Authentic Leaders

- Understand their purpose
- Practice solid values
- Lead with heart
- Establish connected relationships
- Demonstrate self-discipline

—Bill George 2004
"The Journey to Authenticity"

new complaints about parking. In contrast, one patient who is injured in a fall in the bathroom creates a situation that should be analyzed and promptly addressed to assure the highest degree of patient safety.

Learning to identify those critical, differentiating signs requires mindfulness for specific events. Creating focus among the plethora of issues and work to be done in any health-care organization begins with awareness and attention to the point of service, the point of patient care where the fundamental work of the organization occurs. The critical interactions and outcomes of health care occur primarily at the patient-caregiver interaction. Not only must the leader focus on the point of service, and be cognizant of the work of caregivers, the leader must follow the recommendations of direct caregivers. Traditionally, leaders have sought opinions and advice from bedside caregivers, but have not always deferred to them as the ultimate authority. Deferring to the expertise of the provider is much more than recognizing and valuing the opinions of providers, and it is essential for the best processes and solutions.

THE REALITY OF UNCERTAINTY

Vulnerability necessarily leads to uncertainty. There is no roadmap for the future. While the adage "history repeats itself" may be true in some situations and in a rather general way, the reality is that there are no guidelines for the transition from the industrial age to the information age. Some leaders may desire an organization in which employees can be programmed to plod along monotonously and follow established policies, but the events and complexities of patient care render this approach unrealistic. Continuing to work to keep employees in line is futile and frustrating.

Theories within complexity science can assist leaders in creating meaning and understanding of the world as it is, thus mediating some uncertainty. The creation of new pathways for resource use, creation of effective teams, and evaluation of progress become the norm for leaders rather than uncommon events. Specifically, work of complex systems is reflecting the complexity principle that identifies complex systems as being characterized by nonsequential processes that contain many common mode interactions (Zimmerman, Lindberg, & Plsek, 1998). Simple cause and effect is rare indeed. Leaders should expect the unexpected and become wary when the sequence of events becomes predictable.

Mediating Uncertainty: High-Reliability Organizations

The common occurrence of unpredictable challenges places significant demands on leader creativity and imagination. Striving to understand and mediate uncertainty is the most appropriate and logical approach for leaders, rather than working to eliminate variety and hope for stability. Working to achieve stability is irrational given the complex nature of health-care work.

According to Weick & Sutcliffe (2003), recognizing the complex nature of organizations, detecting incredibly weak warning signs, and taking strong decisive action when appropriate are the hallmarks of a high-reliability organization (HRO). HROs have gained credence for their ability to become highly reliable in minimizing errors and thereby increasing patient safety. In addition, HROs have achieved greater stakeholder motivation, time savings, and cost efficiency. These organizations demonstrate the ability to build effective practices and identify unexpected events early on and then respond to these unexpected events in ways that are adaptive rather than destructive. Leaders of HROs thrive in vulnerability, identify different approaches to issues, and take risks in addressing situations in nontraditional ways.

Five characteristics define the high-reliability organization and have direct application to the healthcare industry.

1. *Preoccupation with failure.* The first characteristic of an HRO is preoccupation with failure. In a high-reliability organization, the leader is preoccupied with failure as a means to identify those critical warning signs that signal the need for more examination and quick response. This includes mindfulness to little things, continual scrutiny of the status quo, reviewing expectations, and changing expectations when new information is gained. Minor occurrences are believed to be the precursors of larger, more damaging events.

   In many situations, it is not about how much data is collected or how many questions are asked, but rather what questions are asked about the real-time data that is produced (McGee, 2004). Creating organizational mindfulness to the right signals is about using resources and data effectively. Asking questions that will provide precise and minimum information rather than general aggregated data will avoid an overload of data that must be examined. Leaders need data that will cause them to change a judgment or course of action. For example, if patient feedback data indicates an issue with perceptions of nurses initiating intravenous lines, the issue has specificity and can be quickly investigated and addressed.

   All failures provide insight about the workings of the system. Elaborate screening programs and data-collection processes are in place in most facilities and are intended to probe the vulnerabilities of the organization and learn lessons in order to prevent repetition of costly mistakes. Quality management programs are highly developed, yet these programs are often criticized for failing to identify and address significant errors or sentinel events in a timely manner.

   Further, organizations are challenged to create cultures of safety that support "no-blame" approaches to managing error. Encouraging employees to report even small and inconsequential incidents to facilitate a rapid response for learning and correction can be confused with witch hunting, which focuses on isolating the failure, assigning blame, and never discussing it again. Few failures can be traced to a single individual.

   Interestingly, Weick (Coutu, 2003) tells us that newcomers to an organization are able to identify potential problems and early warning signs more often than experienced, long-term employees. However, new employees are often reluctant to point out problems lest they be identified as troublemakers. Much can be learned from new employees if leaders are able to create cultural expectations that all new employees are required to share such observations at a designated time and without threat of becoming outcasts.

2. *Reluctance to simplify interpretations.* This trait emanates from the tendency to disconfirm evidence that does not meet our expectations. Rather than surrendering to the simplification and standardization of processes, HROs focus on the interactions between people with differing expectations and abilities, which result in different views of the same event. This behavior supports the creation of a safe and respectful environment that allows each person's perspective to be considered and integrated into the work.

   The large volume of procedures performed in health-care organizations necessitates standardized formats and procedures. Yet,

---

Discussion

Creating Mindfulness

1. How mindful is your organization to weak signals?
2. What weak signals have been identified and quickly corrected?
3. What weak signals were missed and resulted in an adverse outcome?
4. Identify new processes to avoid missing a similar signal.

Data Questions in HROs

Ask These Questions:

1. What is the level of patient satisfaction this month?
2. What specific complaints were received this month about specific services?
3. How many new patients used our facilities this month?
4. Are there any supply issues? Has there been a change in product or shortage of needed items?

Avoid These Questions:

1. What real-time information will allow us to detect critical events as quickly as possible—within 1 hour, 2 hours, 24 hours etc.?
2. How can we react faster to negative results?

New Employee Scrutiny

As part of the completion of new orientation, request new members to make three suggestions specific to their ability to do their work based on their initial impressions of the organization.

Discuss the ideas with other members of the team and identify both the advantages and disadvantages of the suggestions.

Should changes be made?

Is it possible to change?

Who will support the changes?

Who will oppose the changes?

What will you do with this information?

patients most likely follow the 80/20 Pareto rule; 80% of patient care can be managed within the standard template while the remaining 20% are anything but routine processes. Simplification of patient care processes using clinical protocols and pathways as the sole determiner of care is potentially dangerous because it limits the precautions individuals take, as well as their ability to envision other deviations that could be harmful.

3. *Sensitivity to operations.* With this trait, leaders believe that expertise resides in those who provide care at the point of service rather than in the executive role. Less bureaucracy, high interaction with caregivers, and sensitivity to the big picture reinforce this sensitivity. This emphasis results in early problem identification and early action.

   Organizational policies are often so well established and followed that the basic work or operations of the facility are compromised. Nearly every valid and well-established policy should be overridden or modified in certain circumstances. The principles of systems theory, in which there are multiple inputs into system operations that use many resources resulting in many differing outputs, can assist individuals in understanding these dynamics.

   Consider the patient with diabetes. The diabetic patient may be an emergency patient, an outpatient, an inpatient, or a surgical patient. Standards of care for diabetic patients are clearly identified for medications, blood glucose monitoring, and skin care. However, in each of the above settings, these standards must be applied within the context of the service in order to achieve the desired outcomes. The standards for blood glucose monitoring instrumentation are applied to the process in each setting using different personnel, different documentation formats, and different feedback mechanisms. Each context requires attention to ensure that standards are met and that the care is individualized to the needs and location of the patient and the standards are met.

   Further, this sensitivity to operations within each setting is expected to support high-reliability organizations. Assuring that blood glucose monitoring is performed accurately and efficiently is an ongoing accountability, no matter how routine the process appears.

4. *Commitment to resilience.* The processes of the health-care system necessarily result in error, due to the human factors of both patients and those providing the care. The expectation for resilience requires new systems and processes to detect and manage errors at the earliest possible stage. According to Weick & Sutcliffe (2001), resilience requires mindfulness about errors that have already occurred and correcting them before they worsen and cause serious harm.

   The notion of error or mistake has resulted in behaviors that seek out the individual responsible for the error and lay blame on the individual. Focusing on resilience begins with a reconceptualization of the concept of error, from a negative event to a reality-based event that did not achieve the intended goals.

   Increasing one's capacity to cope with unanticipated events requires not only a reconceptualization of errors but also preparation for the inevitable surprises by expanding knowledge of new processes of resilience. Creating expectations for thorough and honest evaluation of processes that did not achieve desired goals should become the norm rather than the exception.

5. *Deference to expertise.* HROs develop the ability to alter the traditional deference to status and rank for making decisions in favor of

those who have the expertise to make the decision. The decision makers in HROs are found throughout the ranks of the organization, depending on the issue, accountability, responsibility, uniqueness of the problem, and environmental characteristics.

Traditionally, the executive team has made decisions without the benefit of a clinical perspective, which often results in hindering or delaying patient care. Efforts to minimize such decisions and shift to decisions by experts will necessarily include the complexities of judgment, timing, and team processes and result in more optimal outcomes.

Risk Taking: The Leader's Reputation

Can you afford to make mistakes? Can your organization afford to make mistakes? When is a mistake tolerable? How many mistakes or messages can you make without an impact on your effectiveness? Attention should first be given to the language of mistakes and errors and the existing negative connotations of these words. In order to value information from an unsuccessful attempt, language that is less negative should be considered. Rather than *We cannot afford to have you make a mistake*, questions that are more appropriate for the desired culture of accountability could be used, such as:

- Can you afford to rework your work?
- Can you afford not to rework your work?
- Can the organization afford or expect to rework processes?
- Is it the right thing to do?

Given that life is dynamic and continually evolving, reworking the work and correcting missteps is a responsible leadership behavior. Thus, the answer to these questions is a resounding YES, rework is essential for progress to be made.

When risk taking is spontaneous and haphazard, rather than a systematic process of assessing the situation, weighing alternatives, and taking responsive action based on existing knowledge of the organization and the social, economic, and political context in which it exists, the potential for less-than-satisfactory outcomes and rework increases dramatically. When the leader embraces systematic risk taking, there are no limitations, only expectations for better results.

MEDIATING RISK TAKING

Strategy: Information Management

As organizations adopt more and more computerized management and clinical information systems, data about care proliferates. These technology advances for collecting and managing information bring significant challenges for the leader. Real-time availability of data brings the expectation that leaders will interpret and respond to the data, which is an overwhelming task. The more open the leader is to information, the greater is the expectation for action.

Withholding information in order to sustain power or avoid conflicts is an age-old organizational problem. Recent criticisms of corporate board/CEO-compromised relationships in which CEOs have usurped control from boards through the withholding of information and strong-willed actions are not isolated (George, 2002). Such behaviors are also present throughout the ranks of the health-care organization, from staff nurse to manager to director to executive. Selective information sharing between members of the organization results in less-than-optimal decision making, decreased trust, and poor outcomes.

According to George (2002), creating open communication pathways is about more than good leadership; it is about the legal and fiduciary responsibilities of members of the organization to share the essential information with those accountable for the overall work. Leaders necessarily must be vulnerable in sharing information once believed to be sensitive and must be more open to hearing information that is not positive. Leaders who are not prepared to take the steps to be more open to sharing and receiving all of the pertinent information with the organization should consider leaving the leadership role if they cannot change, rather than compromise the expected governance authority of the organization. All employees are accountable for sharing information about activities that occur, regardless of the perceptions of negativity. Sharing information appropriately is the essence of vulnerability, of openness to others, new ideas, and awareness of limitations.

To shift the power imbalance, clear expectations for communication should be included in job descriptions, as well as a defined review process to ensure objectives are achieved. Once the expectations for information sharing are identified and understood, the next challenge is to ensure that the review process is not a rubber stamp but rather an open, honest, and accurate examination of activities that includes a free flow of ideas and willingness to challenge assumptions and make changes when services can be improved.

Strategy: Embracing Risk

Given that risk taking is an essential behavior in organizations, strategies to thrive as a risk taker are needed. One strategy is to understand and articulate the intangible assets of the organization as a means to guide leaders in determining when and why to take risks. As a result, risk taking can become calculated and focused when consideration is given to three specific types of information: the nature of existing customer relationships, networks of influence, and the information cache within the organization.

Customer relationships include a large number of community members who have frequent and meaningful interactions with the organization, whether through the media, patients, or employees. Health-care organizations also possess detailed knowledge about the community, patients, former patients, and employees and their perceptions of the service provided. Finally, these groups see the health-care organization as the source of expertise. It is respected and trusted.

Networks of relationships exist with key stakeholders such as supply vendors and consultants, who provide valuable insight into the organization. The group of former patients could also be considered as the organization's user group, the group of individuals who use the service and know what works and what does not work for them.

The information owned by a health-care organization is more than the documented patient care information or strategic plan for the future. Knowledge of marketplace activity, technical know-how, financial resources, and by-product information all contribute to the information available to the leaders.

As the leader engages in risk taking, using the available resources about the community, the relationships, and internal information can greatly assist in providing data as to the feasibility of ideas, groups to seek input from, timing within marketplace activities, and overall perceptions of services from multiple stakeholders.

Strategy: Overcoming Silence

Too often leaders are reluctant to express ideas for fear of retaliation or rejection. Past experiences and assumptions about the potential reactions of others render the health-care professional immobile and ineffective.

Leaders must become open and honest in three key situations: sharing opinions and assessments during interview processes, communicating with the media, and providing feedback when negative events occur. Leaders must not only develop competence in these three areas, they must become experts and resources for those with whom they work. Efforts by quantum leaders to reverse the practices of institutionally imposed powerlessness, which expects nurses to not assert themselves individually or collectively, will continue the journey to optimal authenticity. As greater personal and professional authenticity emerges, feelings of low self-esteem, powerlessness, and lack of collegial support can only decrease.

Overcoming this silence leads to increased personal authenticity and greater public awareness of the importance of the role of nurses and all other health-care professionals. Reversing the spiral of silence begins with regular discussions of situations within these three situations, identifying specific events in which silence negatively impacts open and honest communication.

Strategy: Avoiding Risk

In some situations, taking risks is not appropriate, no matter how enticing the idea may be. Any risk that does not support core values, "deprioritizes" the essential responsibilities of the discipline or organization, or provides little return on investment for organizational initiatives should be avoided. Holding to the truth of the work of the healer can only be reflected in unwavering support of value-based quality care that is appropriate to the context of the care and the needs of the patient. When challenging issues are presented, such as the importance of fairness and ethical practices specific to resource allocation, personnel issues, and conflict resolution, the leader must respond with integrity that reflects the authentic self.

Strategy: Reducing Fear

Great decisions bring out the best in teams and further reinforce their ability to achieve greater goals. Yet, typical decision-making team processes often set people against each other. When groups face tough issues, team members with the best of intentions may find themselves locked in divisive and destructive debates. Rather than energizing the processes of teams, this serves to polarize members. Fear, according to Maruska (2004), is the reason. Fear-driven group processes continue because results are generated in many situations. Leaders who have been successful with bullying, threatening tactics do not consider this approach unacceptable; rather, such leaders believe the approach is appropriate because it gener-

---

Discussion

Reversing the Spiral of Silence

Consider the following situations:
- You supported hiring a long-time employee from another department who has a reputation of being very negative.
- Your CEO reacted negatively and aggressively to the press regarding local competition. When asked by the CEO if the communication was distasteful, you respond that it was okay.

What different responses could or should be made to these situations?

What are the risks to you/the organization? The benefits to you/the organization?

Quantum Gem

There is no sin punished more implacably by nature than the sin of resistance to change.

Anne Morrow Lindbergh

The Cycle of Fear Outcomes

1. People get left out of decision making.
2. Participants lost sight of what they really want.
3. Real issues get ignored.
4. Information gathering is biased.
5. Participants are personally attached to preset positions.
6. Decisions don't last.
7. Conflict ensures.

Maruska, 2004

ates results. Unfortunately, while short-term results may be achieved, it is often at the cost of long-term results. Fear-induced behaviors marginalize performance and discourage employees from further meaningful participation in power struggles that are predestined to support the intimidator.

Overcoming the use of fear and shifting to a more collegial environment in which risk taking is valued requires transformation of processes, from motivation by fear to a focus on shared visions, hopes, and dreams. Shifting the focus to shared visions rather than fearful expectations requires a mental model that is much more palatable for teamwork. New behaviors include letting go of personal agendas, a willingness to explore new options that will benefit the team, finding common ground, and creating new, hopeful goals, rather than fear-laden acquiescence to an unsupported solution.

Strategy: Assuring an Ethical Climate

The influence of the workplace on ethical or principled practices is significant, as it may render the leader vulnerable to conflicting peer opinion, loss of colleague approval, physician conflict, and patient dissatisfaction. More often than not, leaders risk changing their relationships and reputation in creating and sustaining an ethical climate.

Many organizational cultures discourage employees from challenging or disagreeing with others and label such behaviors as negative and disruptive. A culture of trust and openness, in which employees are encouraged and expected to identify and confront ethical dilemmas as a team, often requires risk taking in order to make the best decisions and simultaneously value employees.

Employees who participate in decision making and have access to the information necessary to make informed decisions are empowered and contribute significantly to organizational performance. A culture that fosters and reinforces the value of risk-taking behaviors is an essential characteristic of a high-performing organization. The following questions should be considered to ensure ethical decisions:

- Is the action under consideration legal?
- Is the action consistent with organizational policies and guidelines? If not, should a policy be developed?
- Is the action consistent with organizational values?
- Am I personally okay with the proposed action?
- Would I be okay if someone took this action with me?
- Would the most ethical person I know do the same thing?

The diversity of values and beliefs creates a world in which a systematic reflection and analysis of what is right and what is wrong as well as what ought to be done is essential. Ethical issues abound in health-care organizations. The influences of the work setting, demands for greater profits, expectations of safety, and individual motivations require that good and fair decisions are made on a daily basis.

According to Olson (1998), how ethical dilemmas are addressed and the conditions that allow employees to engage in ethical reflection are determinants of the organization's ethical climate. The ethical climate of the organization can either serve to reinforce good and just decisions or to avoid addressing ethical dilemmas, thus blocking healthy dialogue and effective decision making.

While employees should be free to say what is needed about an issue and free to disagree with each other as a means to better understand sit-

---

Key Elements of an Ethical Climate

1. Team members listen to each other.
2. Patients know what to expect.
3. Patients have access to information.
4. Employees believe their manager listens to them.
5. The organization's policies help employees.
6. Nurses believe they practice nursing the way it should be practiced.
7. Conflict is dealt with openly.
8. Nurses and physicians trust one another.
9. Nurses and physicians respect other's decisions.
10. There is a sense of the need for questioning and learning in the organization.

Group Discussion

Consider recent ethical dilemmas that occurred with a peer, manager, physician, or patient.

How was the issue discussed?

When was the issue discussed—close to the event, later, or never?

What should you do in the future to improve the ethical climate of the organization if a similar issue arises?

uations and other perspectives, the organizational culture often does not support or encourage such behaviors. Olson (1998) also suggests that nurses experience the ethical climate through their perceptions of organizational conditions and that practices should present to support the management of difficult patient situations that have ethical implications. How these issues are resolved, whether openly or not at all, reflects the culture support of vulnerable behaviors. Examples of supportive behaviors are listed in Key Elements of Ethical Care.

Strategy: Managing Turnover

The uncertainty of availability of the right individuals to do the work of health care continues to be one of the most significant challenges for the leader. Having the right people to do the job and to do it well is a fundamental expectation for effective leadership. Unfortunately, the rapidly changing environment, cultural mandates, and labor regulations often result in individuals in positions who no longer have the necessary skills for the work of the organization.

To compound the problem, mixed messages are sent to leaders: minimize turnover, maximize productivity, and assure high employee satisfaction. The expectations to be productive and have competent employees become impossible to achieve when some employees have failed to upgrade knowledge and skills and are now not competent to meet the new demands.

According to Waldman, Kelly, Arora & Smith (2004), the average costs to hire and train varies from $3,926 for administrative assistants to $125,543 for attending physicians. These costs associated with turnover raise concerns as to how to manage and decrease the majority of turnover as a cost-savings measure. Two types of turnover are identified in these calculations: healthy turnover and avoidable turnover. It is the avoidable turnover that the leader can positively impact.

Healthy turnover includes a certain number of individuals who are highly mobile and focused on development of skills in a variety of settings, as well as those no longer committed to or supportive of the organization. This turnover is unavoidable and an essential part of organizational life. It is especially true for the individuals of Generations X and Y, who are by nature focused on skill acquisition and personal development rather than loyalty to an organization.

Avoidable turnover results from issues related to health-care policy and practices. Professional disillusionment with the quality of patient care, control over practice, work assignment and schedules, and wage levels can all fuel turnover that may in fact not be necessary. Excessively high rates of turnover of experienced clinicians is more than the cost of doing business. Quality patient care is compromised, the risk of errors increases, morale deteriorates, and overall productivity declines. The quantum leader develops skill in distinguishing avoidable turnover from healthy turnover and focuses on the former.

Strategy: Increase Involvement

The power struggles between all health-care providers, physicians, nurses, therapists, dieticians, social workers, and housekeepers continue to displace the goals of a community of health-care providers learning to live in an age of complexity where goals transcend power struggles. It is ironic that the nursing profession continues to work to empower nursing and to gain autonomy, and yet one of the greatest challenges in health

> ### The Cost of Turnover
>
> The annual cost of turnover (hiring, training, and reduced productivity) represents about 5% of the annual operating budget. Stated differently according to Waldman et al. (2004), it would be revenue neutral to offer each departing nurse (who chose to stay) a staying bonus equal to 86 percent of his or her annual salary or give every nurse on staff a 33% retention supplement every year!
>
> Waldman, Kelly, Arora & Smith, 2004

care is to develop collaborative processes as the means to better patient care. Indeed, it is possible to create and sustain relationships in which the members are both empowered and collaborative.

Leading others is out of date and incongruent with the modern organizational life in the current marketplace. Complexity science proposes a new and better approach than one steeped in autocracy and omniscience. Authority rests in the ability of the leader to see the entirety of the organization and the potential of its people. Quantum leaders cultivate the conditions for the organization to change and grow through the interconnections among people, not through specific individuals using command and control behaviors.

One such way to achieve the new age of leadership is through the leaderless organization concept. The *leaderless organization* makes sense for many reasons, especially since the Internet has dramatically increased the volume and accessibility of information that is available both horizontally and vertically. No longer is information controlled and meted out as the information holder deems appropriate. Allowing or expecting employees to manage themselves can be a significant challenge for the leader. Managing systems and structures of the work context and expecting employees to own the work processes theoretically should lead to better outcomes. Making it a reality requires much more than a declaration of a shared leadership culture.

First, the leader must stop owing every problem and making every decision and must expect that employees are capable—not incapable—of being self-starters, problem solvers, responsible, and independent thinkers. Learning to not only believe that you can trust colleagues but also that you live this belief is essential.

The second strategy in the leaderless organization is to recognize and value the role of the middle manager as an innovator and source of point-of-service information. While this role has indeed evolved considerably over the last ten years, the quantum middle manager is much different from the traditional manager. This role has emerged to be one of both leader and manager, one in which the characteristics of thoroughness, persistence, discretion, persuasiveness, and comfort with change are foundational. Quantum managers' skills are not in being contrary or revolutionary; rather, they are able to work through existing networks, to uncover opportunities, build coalitions, and make change happen. The integration of these skills and competencies into the role of the middle manager serves to further deemphasize command and control while reinforcing openness and valuing of the collective wisdom of the team. The quantum leader is liberated through this complexity approach to leadership and also thrives in the notion that one cannot know or control everything.

MEDIATING RISK

Strategy: Recognizing a Cosmology Episode— The Ultimate Vulnerability

Leaders are often faced with situations in which they believe the universe is no longer a rationale, orderly system, much like the effects of war. Events defy explanation. A cosmology episode, according to Weick (Coutu, 2003), is the opposite of *déjà vu* in which everything suddenly seems familiar and recognizable. In contrast, a state of panic ensues in a cosmology episode and anxiety abounds.

An example of a cosmology episode occurs with the hiring of a new leader. Current employees are faced with a new individual who has significant power over their careers, and yet they have little knowledge of

---

Cosmology Episode

An event or situation in which everything seems strange; a person feels like he has never been here before, has no idea of where he is or who can help him.

Karl Weick, 2003

how the new leader will make decisions, value their role and contributions, and represent them in organizational discussions. Employees have no templates to define what the new leader will do, only uncertainty as to what will happen next. Each new leader brings new values, a new style, and new expectations. While this may not be as dramatic as Weick's hantavirus exemplar of a cosmology episode, such events are occurring more regularly as information technology changes the way work is accomplished (Coutu, 2003). There are fewer and fewer *déjà vu* events and more and more cosmology episodes.

A cosmology episode is impossible to predict. However, some preparation for when it does occur is helpful. Being alert to minor details, avoiding making assumptions until some discussion occurs, reflecting, and working to make sense of what is happening are appropriate behaviors. Weick advises those in cosmology episodes to work hard to transform the raw experience into intelligible world views (Coutu, 2003). Making sense of the cosmology episode lends itself to multiple, conflicting interpretations, all of which may be possible. If an individual or the organization finds itself unsure of where it is going or what it has accomplished, it is essential to be open to many different interpretations. Each action and its consequences assist the leader in editing the list of interpretations down to a manageable set of options. These actions, tempered by reflection, are the critical processes in learning to thrive in a cosmology episode.

STRETCHING

Strategy: Stretching

Taking risks is not the end of the road; it is only the beginning of expanding the capacity of the organization to achieve better results. Stretching one's present skills and abilities to be able to address increasingly difficult situations begins with a strong desire and willingness to move from ordinary solutions to better solutions that improve resource use and clinical outcomes. Quantum leaders provide the vision, which often looks impossible, and continually coach and mentor others to move from novice risk takers to individuals, not only comfortable with risk taking but also able to thrive as risk takers while achieving better outcomes.

Consider the situation in which the leader would like to change the patient care delivery system for several of the patient care units. Stretching would involve not only gaining feedback and support for the new model but also extending the ideas to include more clinical departments, roles, and outcomes. The proposed model can be reviewed with the involved caregivers, as well as former patients, community members, and colleagues in other health-care organizations. Initial feedback can be gained using existing information-gathering networks within the organization and community.

Strategy: Increasing Capacity through Diversity

The complexity of diversity is not always readily apparent. The obvious diversity found in ethnic backgrounds, gender, and age are but the tip of the iceberg. Thinking styles, problem-solving styles, communication styles, decision-making styles, economic status, educational level, and religious affiliation all significantly contribute to organizational complexity and differences within the world of health care. These characteristics are in addition to the plethora of individual values and behaviors.

The fable of the giraffe and the elephant provides an excellent illustration of the multiple realities of the workforce (Thomas & Woodruff,

---

Cosmology Episodes in Your Organization

Just as the switchboard operators and key punch technicians have gone the way of the history books, current health-care procedures are changing quickly and dramatically.

Less invasive procedures, ear temperatures, and computerized documentation all require the elimination of some work in favor of new work.

Identify one procedure/service in your organization that was eliminated last year. What replaced it? How was the new work integrated into the system? Who is now doing new work?

Identify one procedure that you believe will be (or should be) eliminated in the next year. What will replace it? How will the new work be integrated into the system? Who will do the new work?

Gem

Even if it is the harder path, even if it is harder to be true to the self, it is far less painful than being out of step with one's values.

Mary O'Connor, 2003

Diversity

Differences	Similarities
• Skill types	• Health-care workers
• Cultural background	• Share common goals
• Gender	• Work in teams
• Age	• Value relationships
• Values	
• Education level	
• Economic status	

Diversity Maturity Behaviors

- Accept personal responsibility for enhancing personal and organizational effectiveness
- Demonstrate knowledge of self and the organization
- Clear about requirements and decisions about differences and how they impact the ability to meet these requirements
- Understand that diversity is accompanied by complexity and tension and is prepared to cope with these in pursuit of greater diversity effectiveness
- Willing to challenge conventional wisdom
- Engage in continuous learning

R. R. Thomas, 1999,
Building a House for Diversity

Assessing Current Environment Diversity

Identify current processes or services that represent a diversity mixture rather than a "main" and an "other" service.

How did this occur? Why is it sustainable?

Identify processes or services that are based on a "main" group of entity.

Who are the "main" groups? Who are the "others"?

What actions could you take to create a diversity mixture?

What resistance would be encountered?

1999). In this fable, the giraffe builds a house based on the specifications of the giraffe family, which includes high ceilings, narrow doorways, and high windows; the house even wins the National Giraffe Home of the Year Award. In this wonderful house the giraffe has a woodworking shop in the basement. Knowing that his friend from church, the elephant, is also interested in woodworking, he invites the elephant to see his shop and hopes to do work with him in the future. The elephant is delighted and accepts the invitation.

As the elephant attempts to enter the house, he becomes stuck at the front door. The giraffe is not worried because they have installed expandable doors to accommodate wood shop equipment. Once inside the house, the elephant damages the steps to the basement because of his weight and cannot get through the doorway into the shop. The giraffe responds in amazement, then quickly recovers and advises the elephant to join the local gym to slim down and to join a ballet class to become lighter on his feet in order to come into his home.

In this story, the giraffe represents the "main" group; it is his house, his design, his rules, and he is in charge. The elephant represents the "other." While he is warmly welcomed, in the giraffe's house he will always be an outsider since the house was not built with elephants in mind. The story provides a powerful metaphor of traditional attempts to manage diversity and becomes instructive to us in terms of how we really address diversity.

Diversity is a total collective mixture. It is not a function of race or gender or any other us-versus-them dyad, but a complex and ever-changing blend of attributes, behaviors, and talents. A diversity mixture is a combination of individuals who are different in some ways and similar in others.

The process of building a house for diversity is about finding common ground for all and protecting sacred differences. It is not about building a house for one group and making adjustments to accommodate others. Diversity can be seen as a vehicle toward wholeness, a vehicle in which multiple perspectives are held without judgment. Even with the inherent competition of multiple perspectives, the quantum leader understands the value of each perspective and strives to work to acknowledge each contribution, accept the differing perspectives, and integrate them in order to succeed as a team able to recognize and thrive in the collective wisdom produced by the integration of many.

Improving your approach to diversity begins with the recognition of the shortcomings of the traditional approaches of affirmative action, understanding differences, and diversity management.

Affirmative action, which focuses on inclusion and calls for special action to correct the imbalances, does not address the underlying issue of dominant and subordinate factions. For genuine diversity to thrive in organizations, the right climate must be created in which the beliefs and behaviors of all workforce participants are integrated.

Understanding differences is an approach that focuses on relationships and how people get along but does not address structures and organizational policy. There is a reluctance to fully address diversity. The structure or policies represent the needs and values of the main group. The main group identifies differing groups and openly works to acknowledge and accommodate the others. Meeting times, food preferences, and bathroom availability are a few of the typical accommodations made for those with different sleep schedules, cultural food needs, and gender needs.

Finally, the *diversity management* approach proposes to manage or modify the dominant faction to accommodate the subordinate faction. Diversity tension is inevitable. Regardless of how the giraffe's house is modified, it will never be their mutual house. It will remain the house of the giraffe, modified to meet the needs of the elephant. There are no simple solutions with such a complex phenomena except to begin with your internal self and accept personal responsibility for diversity.

Diversity Effectiveness

Creating a climate that integrates and honors differences includes three basic skills and a level of *diversity maturity*. First, it is necessary to identify the differing components that create the diversity and the related tensions that occur. If young and old patients are attending an education program, an understanding of what the differences are is essential. Examples include reading skills, knowledge levels, concentration span, and writing ability, to name a few. Resulting tensions could include length of time for comprehension of content or differing abilities to understand certain terminology.

The second skill is the ability to analyze the mixtures and related tensions. The analysis is performed to identify which differences could interfere with achieving goals. Not all differences need to be addressed if goal attainment is not compromised. If reading time required by one group is twice as long, when does it interfere with goal attainment? If there is only 5 minutes total, no changes need to be made; if there are 30 minutes, changes should be considered to avoid boredom.

The third skill is to select an appropriate response. What should be done regarding the time for comprehension and use of terminology? If the differences are significant, should there be two distinct classes? These three skills are developed with practice and become internalized as core diversity skills to meet leadership challenges.

SUMMARY

Vulnerability continues to be the most significant challenge for leaders in contemporary health-care organizations. Developing not only competence but also expertise in vulnerability behaviors serves the leader in understanding organizational dynamics, appreciating the complexity of relationships and interactions in an organization, and allowing employees to be all that they can be. The strategies to assist leaders in becoming more vulnerable through controlled risk taking will further support the development of expertise. Finally, the incredible power of the five characteristics of a high-reliability organization can be seen as focusing goals for the organization destined to greatness and excellence.

Diversity Effectiveness: Challenges for the Leader

Think about a recent conflict in your work environment.

What diversity components were present? List as many as you can.

Which component(s) interfered with goal attainment?

Consider also:

Did others understand the differences?

Was a lack of trust part of the situation?

Did others have personal agendas?

What will you do differently next time a similar situation occurs?

Exercise 1 Vulnerability and Risk Taking

The current patient care delivery model includes only registered nurses and nursing assistants. The availability of registered nurses and nursing assistants is less than adequate to meet the needs. Your team has examined the situation and is proposing a new patient care delivery model. The model includes roles for master's prepared nurses, baccalaureate nurses, licensed practical nurses, patient care technicians, and certified nursing assistants.

- What risks will you be taking with this proposal?
- What are the goals of this approach? The advantages? The disadvantages?
- How will you mediate the risks?
- What measures will you use to determine the value of the new model?

Exercise 2 High-Reliability Organizations

> The five characteristics of high-reliability organizations have assisted leaders in providing safer, more appropriate patient care services.
>
> In a recent situation, a team made the decision to replace existing blood glucose monitoring equipment in the outpatient, inpatient, surgical, and emergency departments with new equipment that was less costly and believed to be of higher quality in data management. Within two weeks, problems with accuracy and equipment failure were identified in the inpatient and surgical areas. Over 50 patients were identified to have received inappropriate insulin management.
>
> Consider the five principles of a high-reliability organization. Analyze the results in terms of the principles.
>
> Which principles were followed? What changes should be made to improve operations?

REFERENCES

Coutu, D. L. (2003). Sense and reliability: A conversation with celebrated psychologist Karl. E. Weick. *Harvard Business Review* 81(4), 84–90.

George, B. (2004). The journey to authenticity. *Leader to Leader* 31 (Winter), 29–35.

George, W. W. (2002). Imbalance of power. *Harvard Business Review* 80(7), 22–23.

Kellerman, B. (2004). Leadership: Warts and all. *Harvard Business Review* 82(1), 40–45.

Maruska, D. (2004). Making great team decisions. *Leader to Leader* 33(Summer), 38–44.

McGee, K. (2004) Give me that real-time information. *Harvard Business Review* 82(4), 26.

O'Connor, M. (2003). A look at nursing leadership through the lens of a dancer. *Nursing Forum* 38(1), 23–28.

Olson, L. L. (1998). Hospital nurses' perceptions of the ethical climate of their work setting. *Image: Journal of Nursing Scholarship* 30(4), 345–349.

Slywotzky, A. J., & Wise, R. (2002). The growth crisis—and how to escape it. *Harvard Business Review* 80(7), 72–84.

Thomas, R. R., & Woodruff, M. I. (1999). *Building a house for diversity.* New York: AMACOM.

Waldman, J. D., Kelly, F., Arora, S., & Smith, H. L. (2004). The shocking cost of turnover in health care. *Health Care Management Review* 29(1), 2–7.

Weick, K., & Sutcliffe, K. (2001). Managing the unexpected: Assuring high performance in an age of complexity. San Francisco: Jossey-Bass.

Zimmerman, B., Lindberg, C., & Plsek, P. (1998). Irving TX: VHA, Inc.

SUGGESTED READING

Clancy, T. R. (2004). Navigating in a complex nursing world. *JONA* 34(6), 274–282.

DeMarco, R. F., & Roberts, S. J. (2003). Negative behaviors in nursing. *AJN* 103(3), 113–115.

Kanter, R. M. (2004). The middle manager as innovator. *Harvard Business Review* 82(7), 150–161.

Woodburn, L. (2004). Stop leading? *Hospitals & Health Networks* June, 94.

Creating a Culture of Safety

CHAPTER OBJECTIVES:

Upon completion of this chapter, the reader will:

1. Identify the challenges of transforming the organizational health-care culture from one of error avoidance to one in which error is an essential element for improvement.
2. Critique three theories of error and their application to health-care organizations.
3. Translate lessons from the management of clinical errors to the management of errors in leadership.
4. Identify five principles to guide leaders in facilitating the transformation to a culture of safety.

INTRODUCTION

Traditional society values success and provides winners with recognition, trophies, financial rewards, and promotions. The achievement of goals and best practices receives high recognition while leadership failure is more likely recognized as a scarlet letter, or worse, is not discussed at all. Yet, along the journey to success, leaders do indeed experience failures or less positive than anticipated results. Failure is bound to occur in every organization and in every career.

A new perspective is needed in order to recognize and value the information gained in less than successful attempts. Leaders need to reverse many assumptions and learn to embrace situations in which the desired outcomes were not realized. Failures must be viewed as acts of courage and recognized as essential behaviors that do indeed support a culture of excellence for the incredible insight and dialogue that results. A positive and realistic interpretation of the failure experience and the resulting lessons provides all leaders with necessary experiences for a better future. This chapter presents an overview of theories of error, the characteristics of the current health-care culture of error avoidance, and strategies to transform the health-care culture to one that values errors

> **Failures & Mistakes are . . .**
> - Lack of success, a deficiency, or falling short
> - Not achieving something desired
> - Portals of discovery (James Joyce)
> - The highway to success, as each discovery of what is false leads us to seek earnestly after what is true. (John Keats)

as opportunities. Five principles to guide the transformation are presented to assist leaders in this important journey.

A perspective grounded in valuing the experience of error begins with the transition from *discipline* as the initial reaction to *remediation,* in which the human factors are identified and an effort to learn from error events is an expectation rather than an option.

THEORIES OF ERROR

Errors are defined in numerous ways, most of which reflect failures or unwanted outcomes. Failures, according to Leape (1999) have been described in two categories: *active* or system errors that stem from characteristics of communication systems, job design, or equipment, and *latent* or organizational failures that arise from decisions made by people with indirect responsibilities. Both accidents and recurrent errors result from a series of human decisions associated with both active and latent failures, with active failures having the more immediate and obvious consequences and latent failures undermining organizational efforts to create a safe environment.

Error as Foolishness

Given the reality of human nature and its normal state of imperfection, some scholars have attempted to explain error from an interesting perspective of errors as the result of human foolishness (Kaye, 2000). Humanity begins in a state of perfection, and the journey of life is filled with temptation and distractions. Understandably, humanity partakes from the tree of information and experience that includes both good and evil.

As people mature and stray from the initial state of perfection, errors or mistakes are made. People become distracted and tempted by many things, often the desire for more worldly goods. Not surprising, people follow their desires, losing the awareness of perfection, ignoring the inner voice of wisdom, and giving into the temptation. Sometimes, individuals risk everything for one more personal thing—another automobile, boat, computer, or vacation—negating the sense of personal wholeness. Error results.

While not all leaders may be comfortable with the theory of errors as foolishness, this mental model provides a framework from which to examine the phenomena of errors in a more positive way, one that humanizes the error factor. Recognizing that mistakes are expressions of inescapable foolishness rather than the result of malice enables individuals to let the errors go and to avoid taking them personally so that they do not cast a shadow over a lifetime's career.

Accepting ourselves and our own mistakes in this way can serve as the basis for responding to the mistakes of others with understanding, rather than responding with anger and resentment (Porter-O'Grady & Malloch, 2003).

Further, the errors as foolishness perspective allows individuals to overcome the human tendency to hold a grudge when an error is made that is believed unnecessary and avoidable. Quantum leaders learn to forgive others when a mistake is made and begin to coach others to learn from the event. Moving beyond the resentment of grudges encourages others to expect to be treated as others treat them, with understanding and kindness. Now the leader can move from the need for punishment as the rem-

> Failure IS an option . . . when you are dealing with human reality!

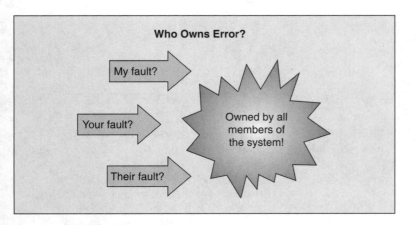

Who Owns Error?

My fault?

Your fault?

Their fault?

Owned by all members of the system!

edy to error to a new mental model in which error is an opportunity for growth. Learning to believe and trust that mistakes may in fact bring great fortune and new opportunities is the only way to move from the toxicity of a blameful culture to one of accountability.

Sagan (1993) identified two theories of error: normal accident theory and high reliability theory. Each theory reflects differing assumptions specific to the basic nature of how organizations operate and analyze complex situations.

Normal Accident Theory

The basic assumption of normal accident theory is that accidents are inevitable in complex systems. In many ways, there is a contradiction to decision-making philosophy: Decentralization is needed to manage the complexity of the system and centralization is expected to assure tight controls and standardization. System redundancy is believed to be the cause of accidents and further increases interactive complexity and encourages inappropriate risk taking. The theory is similar to a military model that includes strong discipline and control, which is much different than a model of shared leadership and collaborative decision making. There is no way that organizations can train for unanticipated, dangerous, or politically unacceptable situations within this theoretical framework. Finally, the most problematic notions of this theory include the denial of personal responsibility, faulty reporting, and the negative value of reviewing error incidents.

High Reliability Theory

In contrast, high reliability theory assumes that intelligent organizational design and management can avert serious errors when four factors are integrated in the system: safety as a priority; high redundancy in both technical and personnel systems; decentralized operations; and well-developed trial-and-error organizational learning processes. The core belief of this theory is that accidents or errors can be prevented though good organizational design and management. Redundancy enhances safety, as duplication and overlap can render a system reliable rather than unreliable. Continuous evaluation, training, and simulations further support and maintain high-reliability operations. And most importantly, trial-and-error learning from accidents is believed effective and necessary.

THE CULTURE OF ERROR AVOIDANCE

Each of these perspectives offers insight into the existing health-care culture of organizational error avoidance. The health-care culture is embedded with complex communication processes and conflicting values. Within most health-care organizations, unique social hierarchies are dominated by the medical profession. This long-standing social stratification has a profound impact upon the relationships, communication practices, conflict management, expectations for collaboration, displays of emotion, and patient care practices. Dominance of one group over another has contributed significantly to the prevailing practices that support error avoidance and further darken the landscape of error management and the resulting disciplinary processes.

Efforts to address the dark side of discipline require a strong organizational culture that encourages and values safety, accountability, and empowerment of employees to perform responsibly rather than robotically. Standards are necessary for order and consistency but are seldom

---

Discussion

Three theories of error, error as foolishness, normal accidents, and high reliability, provide the foundational philosophy for much error management.

- Which theory does your organization or department subscribe to?
- How was this choice made?
- Is there a need for a theoretical shift in thinking?
- How would this shift be accomplished?
- Who would be involved?
- Who are the supporters?
- What are the barriers?

High-Reliability Organizations' Defining Characteristics

1. Preoccupation with failure
2. Reluctance to simplify work
3. Sensitivity to operations
4. Commitment to resilience
5. Deference to expertise

Weick & Sutcliffe, 2001

Culture

The integrated pattern of human knowledge, belief, and behavior that depends upon man's capacity for learning and transmitting knowledge to succeeding generations.

Merriam-Webster's Dictionary

Common Expressions of Culture

- Observed regularities: how people interact, their language, customs, and traditions
- Group norms: implicit standards and values, such as meetings always starting on time
- Espoused values: the publicly announced principles that the group claims to be trying to achieve
- Formal philosophy: the broad policies and ideological principles that guide a group's actions toward employees, customers, and stakeholders
- Climate: the feeling that is conveyed in a group by the physical layout and the way in which members of the organization interact with each other, with customers, and with outsiders
- Embedded skills: the special competencies group members display in accomplishing certain tasks
- Rules of the game: the implicit rules for getting along in the organization that a newcomer must learn to become an accepted member
- Habits of thinking, mental models: the shared cognitive frames that guide the perceptions, thought, and language used by the members of the group
- Shared meanings: the emergent understandings that are created by group members as they interact with each other
- Integrating symbols: the ideas, feelings, and images groups develop to characterize themselves, which may or may not be appreciated consciously but become embodied in buildings, office layout, and other material artifacts of the group

Root Cause Analysis: Facilitator or Barrier?

If unwanted situations tends to occur repeatedly, then it might be beneficial to figure out what is really causing this situation to occur and remove it so the situation does not occur again. This process, root cause analysis, involves finding the real cause of the problem and dealing with it rather than simply continuing to deal with the symptoms and has become commonplace in health care.

But is "root cause analysis" really an appropriate phrase and approach when our world is endlessly interconnected and everything seems to influence so many other things? Seeking the "root cause" may be a reinforcement of a culture focused on finding blame rather than one supporting error as opportunity. Do you agree? Disagree?

appropriate for all situations, as the reason for ongoing human evaluation and modification of standards is to assure that the evolving goals of safety and quality are indeed met.

Within the current culture of error avoidance four common themes have been identified as contributing to the situation: first, longstanding problems that have not been addressed; second, the potential harm was significant; third, the management systems were inadequate; and fourth, little was learned by leaders from repeated errors. Another confounding issue is that time for learning and remediation of systems has been limited or nonexistent in financially strapped organizations. Additionally, the failure to learn from errors is often not caused by the lack of interest in learning to improve processes, but rather is the result of the strong disincentives against exposing serious failures. The two sets of records (external and internal documents) further constrain learning opportunities. Interestingly, efforts to internally examine what really occurred and to fully discuss the situation often result in "transforming" the experiences of failure into successes as a means to mediate liability! [No changes in unsafe systems or behaviors occur to decrease liability exposure.]

Finally, while the attempt to analyze errors through sentinel events and root cause analysis (RCA) has increased awareness and focus on significant errors, the limitations of the RCA are problematic. Few problems can be traced to a single or root cause; most problems or errors are the result of multiple factors in the environment and multiple interactions between multiple providers (Scott, 2004). The RCA is only the beginning step of error analysis, not the end point.

TRANSFORMING THE HEALTH-CARE CULTURE

Leaders are called to create better systems for investigating failures, reporting errors, and for implementing the lessons learned. Eliminating practices that support secrecy, defensiveness, and deference to authority is essential in transforming the current health-care culture. The next step is to create strong incentives for reporting errors and to support the identification of failures as means to work more effectively.

A culture supportive of safety requires a compelling vision related to patient safety, structures to oversee patient safety and the cultural evolution, systematic approaches to examining and addressing errors, practice and support for team learning, and reinforcement of new behaviors. To begin the journey, much can be learned from clinical error research.

LESSONS FROM CLINICAL ERROR MANAGEMENT

Clinical errors have been analyzed extensively in the recent past and offer information not only about the error but also about the systems in which the errors occur. The clinical errors that have been studied include unnecessary procedures, treatment complications, and near-miss situations. Fortunately, recommendations from the Institute of Medicine (2001) and Page (2004) have identified many of the specific actions that can improve patient safety. However, overall the analyses provide information that is both alarming and challenging. According to Walshe & Shortell (2004), in most cases of major failure the systems of quality management in health-care organizations have been unable to cope with the identified problems. Current systems intended to manage clinical errors are easily bypassed or sidetracked and fail to raise the alarm that something is wrong.

The recommendations from clinical error experiences require changes in not only the culture of the organization but also in leader behaviors for initiating and sustaining practices supportive of patient safety. Error events occur in the processes of leadership as well as in the provision of patient care. For the most part, it is only the leader or the team of individuals responsible for the context of care that can change conditions to minimize both leadership and clinical error as the vehicle to improving patient safety. Given the many perspectives and complex dynamics within the error event, this task is no small challenge.

Leaders need to translate the processes and lessons learned from the analysis of clinical errors and facilitate the needed cultural changes to create the desired culture of safety. They must also examine their own failed practices to provide more reliable systems. Gaining an understanding of fundamental error research, assessing one's organization, creating principles of leadership safety, and facilitating the necessary changes to transform the cultures are all necessary steps in the journey to excellence.

LEADERSHIP ERROR

Unlike clinical error, leadership error is largely uncharted territory in health-care literature (Chaffee & Arthur, 2002). Many interpretations of leadership error exist and traditionally focus on the failure to deliver health-care services, the mismatch between an individual and the work to be done, or inadequate educational preparation. Regardless of the perspective of leadership error, a new lens that expects leaders to focus on learning from the experience of the error rather than attempting to eliminate errors is essential in the journey to excellence.

Many lessons can be learned from the recent studies on clinical patient safety. The solutions to problems that address the interwoven contributions of both the individual and the established collective culture of an organization have not been readily apparent. While it often seems straightforward to affix blame to either the individual or the system, solutions that exclusively focus either on the individual or on the organization have been less than acceptable to the health-care industry. A shift from an error mentality that requires punishment to a mindset that values error as opportunity and includes the realities of human factors such as the amount and type of experience, level of skill, level of fatigue, and motivation affecting a person's ability to perform well is essential in order for progress to be made.

The National Council of State Boards of Nursing's seminal work in the study of registered nurse discipline is the Taxonomy of Root Cause Analysis Protocol (TERCAP). Several categories are relevant in the study of leadership error and include initial human factors consideration. The TERCAP categories of lack of attentiveness, lack of professional accountability, inappropriate judgment, poor judgment in the supervision of others, and documentation errors will be presented as vehicles in the creation of leadership safety principles.

ONE IMPORTANT CAVEAT: CULT OR CULTURE FOR TRANSFORMATION

First and foremost, the need for transformation from a punitive culture to an error-supportive culture is not an option. The health-care industry cannot afford to shield and avoid the reality of errors. Further, it is not a choice about changing policies and report formats to external agencies; it is an expectation from consumers and requires an understanding of the organizational culture and how to effectively begin the

---

Essential Elements for Cultural Transformation

- A vision that identifies safety as a priority
- Commitment to replacing systems that don't work
- Support for continuous learning of all employees to strengthen the system
- Resources within the organization to expect, support, and reward critical thinking

---

Leadership Failure

- Failure to achieve a specific, defined organizational goal as a result of intrinsic (errors made by the leader in planning or execution) or extrinsic (system factors not within the leader's sphere of influence) factors.
- The inability to exhibit basic leadership skills of enabling others to do their work, role modeling, challenging processes, and inspiring a shared vision.

Human Factors

- Motivation
- Skill level
- Experience
- Fatigue

Human Factors

- The discipline that tries to optimize the relationship between technology and the human (Kantowitz and Sorkin, 1983).
- The central approach of human factors is the application of relevant information about human characteristics and behavior to the design of objects, facilities, and environments that people use (Grandjean, 1980).
- The goal of human factors is to apply knowledge in designing systems that work, accommodating the limits of human performance and exploring the advantages of the human operator in the process (Wickens, 1984).
- Human factors discovers and applies information about human behavior, abilities, limitations, and other characteristics to the design of tools, machines, systems, tasks, jobs, and environments for productive, safe, comfortable, and effective human use (Chapanis, 1985).

Taxonomy of Error Root Cause Analysis Protocol Categories (TERCAP)

- Lack of attentiveness/surveillance
- Lack of or faulty intervention
- Lack of professional accountability
- Inappropriate judgment
- Missed or mistaken order
- Lack of prevention
- Documentation errors
- Medication errors

Benner, Sheets, Uris, Malloch, Schewd & Jamison, 2003

Personal Cult vs. Culture

A rudimentary, incomplete, inherently ephemeral phenomenon that fades away when the personality that creates it departs. In contrast, a culture is much more durable and robust than a cult, because its survival and strength do not require the presence and personality of a single individual.

Deering, Dilts & Russell, 2003

Self-Awareness Assessment

- Do I view failure as a personal flaw?
- Do I view failure as the outcome of many factors, individuals, and expectations?
- Am I comfortable in addressing failure as a means to increase the organization's ability to move forward?
- Do I overemphasize my strengths at the expense of weaknesses?
- How did I react to:
  - The last error in budget management?
  - Negative patient outcome?
  - Failure to achieve competency?
  - Hiring of an individual who did not have expected competencies?

---

long and arduous journey in changing fundamental behaviors, beliefs, and values. Such a journey will not occur quickly or without significant struggle, even though most leaders know in their heart that it should be done quickly and with the support of all of the industry.

The journey to a culture of safety requires more changes in behavior than most can envision initially. The transformation must be focused on sustainable cultural change rather than superficial behavior changes that are strongly supported by the leader and champion for safety. Leaders are expected to add value to the organization that is sustainable long after they leave.

Creating a culture of leadership requires the leader to plan to become indispensable as the culture permeates the organization. According to Deering, Dilts, & Russell (2003), if an organization falls apart after the leader departs, the subsequent ruin is, in a sense, a validation of the leader's talent and evidence of the value added during his or her tenure. It is also evidence of the leader's failure to endow the organization with the qualities needed to transcend previous achievements and nurture the conditions under which leadership can exist successfully.

Some leaders unknowingly fail to create a culture of leadership and instead foster a personal *cult*—a rudimentary, incomplete, inherently ephemeral phenomenon that fades away when the personality who created it departs. In contrast, a culture is much more durable and robust, because its survival and strength do not require the presence and personality of a single individual. Culture is something that arises from and is shared by all members of an organization or social system. Organizations with leadership cultures will outperform leadership cults in the following three aspects: anticipating what is needed, aligning values and behaviors, and acting on the basis of priorities that will sustain the culture. Given this, the message is clear to leaders as they embark on changing the current health-care culture. As leaders facilitate the transformation to a culture in which error is valued as an opportunity, the risk of creating a cult is significant. Too often, changes are viewed as fads and attached to specific individuals rather than integrated into the essential core of the culture. Avoiding creation of a cult in favor of a long-standing sustainable culture will support the organization rather than render it sensitive to each new superficial fad designed to improve safety.

CREATING A CULTURE OF SAFETY: FIVE PRINCIPLES FOR LEADERS

Transformation of the health-care culture requires commitment, a clear and compelling vision, and guiding principles to support progress and serve as checkpoints for evaluation. The following five principles are offered to the leader and are based on current research and publications specific to error research, cultural transformation, and contemporary leadership in complex systems. Each principle includes an overview of the principle, non-supporting behaviors that should be changed, and supportive strategies to strengthen the processes of cultural transformation.

Principle #1. Self-Awareness of Leadership Style, Values, and Beliefs

The first principle is self-awareness of one's leadership style, values, and beliefs. Knowing your values and reactions to clinical error or any failure within the organization is the first and most important step in cultural transformation. Indeed, personal awareness requires careful analysis of how errors are acknowledged, discussed, and documented. For most leaders, a new lens from which to understand failure is needed. While most leaders know that failure of some type at some level is a fact of life, the ambivalence about failure has created an unhealthy state of denial that begins with individual values and perceptions of error as failure that cannot be tolerated and must be eliminated. Our hearts know that failure is inevitable, yet our heads too often tell us that punishment is an essential and expected leader behavior.

Learning to view failure as the result of many factors rather than personal inadequacy is much easier said than done. Working with colleagues to change behaviors and attitudes, acting as coaches and mentors for each other, is the first step in the transformation. Informal, ongoing commitment to new behaviors creates more sustainable change than a one-day seminar. Working in small groups to critique and reinforce each other supports timely dialogue and minimizes the fear of intimidation. Further, leader colleagues can address the unrealistic expectations for performance, assure that adequate time is taken to reflect on one's personal impact and progress in changing behavior, and recognize successful encounters with error.

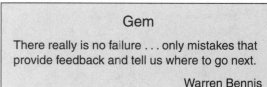

> ### Gem
>
> There really is no failure . . . only mistakes that provide feedback and tell us where to go next.
>
> Warren Bennis

Poor Judgment in the Supervision of Others

A common leadership error involves poor judgment in the supervision of others. The error could be the result of over-, under- or inadequate supervision. The span of control for leaders may become unmanageable with overwhelming numbers of individuals to facilitate, leaving many gaps in the key processes of health-care work. Not knowing what is occurring, it cannot be monitored or modified. This is not to imply that micromanagement is necessary to be sure that everything is done correctly, but leaders need to be cognizant of the real-time effectiveness of processes and be able to *course correct* as quickly as possible when indicated.

Another example of poor judgment in the supervision of others is the inappropriate assignment of duties to colleagues or managers that is beyond their scope of competence, experience, or communication skills. The situation is further compromised when expectations are not clearly communicated, leaving the individual at risk for failure given that the expectations are not identified. Consider the situation in which an executive requests a newly hired director to attend a physician meeting in his or her place without clear expectations. The director, new to the organization, is unaware of the meeting agenda protocols, personalities of the attending members, and the role of an ex-officio. While the director will eventually be quite competent to attend meetings in place of the executive, this situation could quickly become a negative experience and require significant efforts to reverse the impressions of both the new employee and members of the committee. If the new employee interacts without background information.

Another example of poor judgment in the supervision of others is inadequate or infrequent monitoring of manager performance and outcomes. While the leader may be aware of the long hours put in by the director and assume that goals are being accomplished, failure by the leader to review outcomes regularly may reveal little or no progress when a review is actually held. The manager has indeed been physically present in the facility, but not engaged in work expected for the role. Both the leader and the director are disappointed and frustrated as both assumed progress was being made. Poor judgment was made in assuming that work was being accomplished by the mere presence of the director in the facility. In essence, the leader delegated appropriately but

> ### Leadership Error
>
> **Inappropriate Judgment Examples**
>
> - Staff abandonment in times of great uncertainty and risk
> - Failure to act due to reimbursement
> - Inappropriate priorities (tunnel vision)
> - Inappropriate withholding of resources
> - Inappropriate acceptance of delegation/assignment

> ### Leadership Error
>
> **Lack of Professional Accountability Examples**
>
> - Lack of respect for staff concerns and dignity
> - Attributes responsibility to others (lack of integrity)

did not effectively supervise the assignment and was unknowingly directing substandard care processes.

Strategy: Be Accountable

Increasing professional accountability is an important step in addressing poor judgment issues. The lack of fiduciary or professional accountability has been identified (Benner, Sheets, Uris, Malloch, Schwed & Jamison, 2002) as a significant factor in error events. Leaders are expected to create and support the infrastructure for a culture of professional and personal accountability that includes behaviors, organizational norms, and management practices. The culture must eliminate or at least minimize those behaviors that reflect avoidance of accountability and reinforce behaviors supportive of accountability. Several behaviors are identified as not supportive leader actions:

- Failing to put the organization (mission, values, beliefs) first
- Ignoring staff concerns or requests due to time, schedule, resources or existing policy; denying accountability; delayed decision making in hopes of system self-correction
- Misunderstanding or violating the leader-staff-patient relationship; pointing the finger at others; claiming confusion and lack of understanding or information from recent meetings/communication
- Not acting responsibly in protecting staff, patient, family and community vulnerabilities; supports physician abuse or poor staffing in favor of controlling expenses and maintaining revenues
- Not notifying others of significant events that impact the reputation and operations of the organization; fearful of feedback
- Lack of insight regarding staff needs; lack of sensitivity to differing generational and diversity needs; behaviors steeped in the values of one generation rather than multiple, diverse needs

Reversing these ineffective behaviors begins with a personal assessment of leadership style and adopting the following behaviors:

- Own your own circumstances and the results achieved. Solutions come only after someone takes the initiative to explore, search, and ask questions.
- Stay engaged. Commit yourself 100% to the work at hand. When difficult challenges persist, it is easy to give up and stop trying or to wait and see if things will get better on their own. Avoid this trap and consider what CAN be done instead of what CANNOT be done.
- Recognize the full reality of the situation and the contributions of multiple individuals. Create new relationships that involve others you may not have previously considered to be a part of the solution.
- Challenge current assumptions to support the best processes and outcomes. Be persistent in formulating new and creative solutions that make progress possible.
- Avoid wasting time and energy on things you cannot change. Acknowledge the reality of problems and challenges.
- Just do it, even if it is difficult.
- Never fear learning from your mistakes!

Principle #2. Plan for Errors

Effective planning for error is about error prevention. That requires leaders assume very little, decrease their reliance on memory, and learn

---

Leadership Error

Faulty Intervention Examples

- Deliberate error cover-up or avoidance of the issue
- Boundary violations, for example, over-modifies policies for selected employees based on personal relationships
- Breach of confidentiality
- Fails to detect faulty or missing information (lack of critical analysis)
- Initiates new programs without adequate orientation or training

to develop cues that increase awareness of potential problems. The leader must increase awareness for minor but critical signals.

While it is impossible to prevent all errors, it is possible to be more prepared for the future. Reducing the risk of failure is a critical leadership behavior, and this includes the ability to define what might happen in the future and choose among available alternatives as a means to mediate risk. Leaders are challenged to create an infrastructure that will support early identification and open discussion of errors, in order to create better processes that will lead to fewer opportunities for errors and better patient outcomes. Learning to control the areas over which one has control and minimizing the areas in which there is little control is a relatively new mindset for the quantum leader. Equally important is the need for the leader to not become risk intolerant but to be able to recognize and tolerate enough risk to assure quality and progress into the future, an often difficult position to determine. The level of risk tolerance that the leader selects is necessarily related to the significance of the potential undesirable outcomes.

Nonsupporting behaviors are reflected in the leader's lack of attentiveness to the needs of employees, to the results of ineffective systems, and to the lack of appropriate caregiver skills. In essence, the leader does not know which signposts or events within system processes are critical and require monitoring and intervention. This is different from willful neglect of duty; it is a lack of knowledge about what to observe and what to do. How employees are performing, their level of satisfaction and morale, and the level of clinical outcome achievement are essential variables that require monitoring. In essence, this leader is unaware of the system needs and unable to develop proactive plans to support positive error management systems.

Strategy: Plan for Error Communication

A very important expectation for the leader in planning for errors is to create communication processes and expectations that allow for timely discussion of error-related issues. The agenda for such a discussion should include a review of overall results, reinforcement of good judgment, identification of situations in which near misses or failure to rescue was identified, solutions to identified problems, and review of the appropriate documentation needed. Participation in error discussion must include those responsible for and involved in the outcome to minimize handoff or communication delays. Limiting discussion to leaders and excluding direct caregivers decreases the potential for timely and comprehensive review of situations, development of appropriate solutions, and support from those responsible for implementing the new interventions. Finally, back-up or alternate mechanisms for communication need to be created by the leader to assure that caregivers have timely access to discussion and solutions.

Assuring access to information as well as discussion is also significant for an effective process. Individuals need access to both electronic and paper data as a support for timeliness and quality. Communication of information should include multiple communication modalities: electronic, paper, and face-to-face sharing of information, not one modality exclusively. Using e-mail and the Internet are adjuncts to good face-to-face dialogue, not replacements. Finally, back-up or downtime systems for electronic processes need to be established for timely resolution of issues.

Strategy: Managing Professional Licensure

Many caregivers hold professional licenses; physicians, nurses, pharmacists, and therapists. While less than 2% of licensees are brought to a

---

Gem

If you drop a frog into a pan of hot water, the frog will immediately react to the heat by jumping out of the pan. But, if you carefully place the same frog in a pan of comfortably cold water, then slowly raise the temperature, the frog will accept the change, and perhaps without noticing it, stay in the water until the heat kills it.

We all run the risk of getting cooked if we fail to notice the small changes that take place around us.

professional board for discipline, the occurrence of board violations is traumatic to both the organization and the individual.

Quantum leaders develop proactive processes to assure safe and legal practice by providers, and they work to decrease the potential for practice act violations. Developing specific plans to inform license holders of the specific state practice acts and the most common discipline categories is an example of a proactive step to assist practitioners to practice within the law. Approaches that support a proactive approach rather than a reactive approach can increase job satisfaction, reinforce the importance of safe staffing, and minimize situations that require reporting to the professional board.

Review of license scopes of practice and violations is best accomplished as part of new employee orientation and during annual updates. This approach serves to position employees for success, reinforces the legitimate role of the practitioner, and minimizes the potential for violations of professional practice acts. Discussion of multiple roles as a matrix of role accountabilities that identifies role boundaries is a valuable exercise in reinforcing expectations for practice. Discussion of the common licensure violations provides specific information and situations for employees to assist them to avoid such behaviors, a proactive approach. Sharing both the specific role accountabilities and the common deviations raises employee sensitivity to vulnerable situations and decreases opportunities for licensure violations. Examples of violations of licensure nurse practice acts in which nurses are disciplined include the following:

- Practicing beyond scope
- Medication errors
- Falsification on employment application
- Alcohol abuse
- Drug abuse/drug diversion
- Positive drug screen
- Failure to supervise
- Failure to assess and intervene
- Sexual misconduct
- Leaving duty station
- Theft from employer
- Theft from patient
- Documentation errors

Strategy: Assure Safe Staffing

An element of safe staffing is the number of hours that caregivers are scheduled to work. Recent research (Rogers, Hwang, Scott, Aiken & Dinges, 2004) suggests that the use of extended work shifts and overtime has escalated as hospitals try to cope with the shortage of nurses. The evidence in this first national effort to quantify hospital staff nurse work hours and work patterns and the relationship to errors and near errors is significant, according to Rogers and colleagues (2004). The risk of making an error significantly increased when work shifts were longer than 12 hours, when nurses worked overtime, or when they worked more than 40 hours per week. The real challenge for leaders becomes one of recognizing and evaluating the impact of this research on current staffing patterns, error rates, and staff availability. No simple solutions to this challenge are on the horizon.

Strategy: Rework the Physical Environment

Several key variables in the work environment have been identified as negatively impacting staff stress levels and increasing patient care errors. Leader involvement in design and redesign of the physical environment for patient care has never been more critical. Design of both work processes and workspaces can decrease medication errors and nosocomial infections. The most notable feature in reducing errors in the design of patient physical space is the provision of single-bed patient rooms rather than multiple-bed rooms or wards (Page, 2004).

The availability of reference material for nurses, unit dose dispensing, barcoding of medications, and smart infusion pumps, as well as physical space for medication preparation that is isolated to minimize distractions (no phone in the medication room) and adequate lighting are features that leaders should assure are present in the work setting (Page, 2004; Ulrich, Quan, Zimring, Joseph, & Choudhary, 2004). The recent review of over 600 rigorous research articles by Ulrich et al. (2004) is required reading for leaders who are focused on the physical environment as an important consideration in creating safer built environments for health-care services.

Strategy: Reduce Handoffs

The transfer or handoff of patients from nurse to nurse, shift to shift, unit to unit, and organization to organization has been identified by Cook, Render & Woods (2000) as a potential source of errors and adverse patient outcomes. Many errors originate from slips in transfers of materials, information, instructions, and different individuals. Armed with this information, leaders are well positioned to contribute to the planning for new or redesigned physical spaces and work processes, given that the gaps created during the handoff processes are known to threaten patient safety and waste resources.

Strategy: Better Project Management

Many organizations have become quite competent in the management of projects and integration of sophisticated project management methodologies. Yet, not all projects are successful; some lead to unanticipated and undesired results. When good projects fail, chances are the idea was good but the process of implementation was flawed. Project plans, timelines, and budgets are established to reduce the execution risk, which is the risk that the necessary activities will not be carried out properly. Plans are monitored carefully and systematically. Project teams execute their tasks on time and under budget, and yet the overall project still may fail to deliver the intended results. According to Matta and Ashkenas (2003), two critical risks are often neglected; the "white space risk" that some required activities won't be identified in advance, leaving gaps in the project plan, and the "integration risk" that the disparate activities won't come together at the end.

Several strategies can be used to avoid project failures.

- Focus on results first, processes of project management second
- Challenge the assumptions to be sure the "white space" or the unknowns are identified as quickly as possible throughout the project. Ask questions such as "Who else cares about this work?" and "Is there someone that can enhance or will challenge this work?"

The Cost of Patient Handoffs

1. Potential delays in treatment. The average time from transfer order to arrival in new room is 5.1 hours
2. Average cost of labor per transport: $35.17/hour
3. Indirect costs of lost productivity, transport equipment, duplication and rework of patient care documentation, additional linen and housekeeping expenses
4. An increase of 0.5 days in hospital stay due to disruptions in the care processes

Cook, Render & Woods, 2000

White Space

Examples of white space include:

- Hidden financial costs
- Unknown competing projects
- New legislative mandates
- Unknown project resistors

The Ultimate Dilemma: Standardize or Personalize?

Consider the situation of medication administration. The clinical staff has determined that all medications will be passed at standardized times to assure completion of the task and decrease errors of omission. Recently, patients have requested to take medications at different times more like their own medication times at home.

- How will you address this situation?
- What are the advantages and disadvantages of each approach?
- What changes should or should not be made?
- What is the rationale for your changes and how will you monitor the results?

Research Utilization

The use of knowledge typically based on a single study.

Barnsteiner & Prevost, 2002

Evidence-Based Practice

The conscientious use of current best evidence in making decision about patient care. It integrates:

- A systematic search for and critical appraisal of the most relevant evidence specific to a clinical question
- One's own clinical experience
- Patient preferences and values

Sackett, Straus, Richardson, Rosenberg & Haynes, 2000

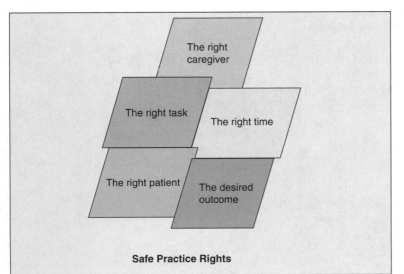

Safe Practice Rights

- Recognize that it is not possible to identify, plan for, and influence all of the variables in advance; what can be done is the creation of processes to continually challenge the assumptions and having the willingness to modify processes to achieve goals.

Principle #3. Create Balance between Standardization and Customization

The Catch-22 of health care must certainly be the need for standardization of processes to achieve reliability and personalization of care to support patient involvement and satisfaction! How does the leader assure consistent processes and still support patient care that considers the diverse values, beliefs, age, education, and culture of each individual? Mandates from regulatory agencies, accrediting organizations, and professional licensing boards require leaders to create policies supportive of safe practices, clinical standards, and fiscal viability. Coupled with these mandates is the expectation that leaders also create the organizational context that supports personalization of health care. Necessarily, given the complex and multiple accountabilities of the leader, work should be designed to minimize the need for human tasks that are known to be especially fallible. Checklists, protocols, and computerized decision tools should be incorporated whenever possible.

Strategy: Evidence-based Practice

Standardization based on personal agendas and opinions rather than evidence and rationale has resulted in significant redundancies in health care. While there has never been an excess of resources for health care, practice has not been focused on evidence until more recently. Efforts to become more judicious in the use of limited resources have elevated the need for evidence-based practices. Thus, it is through the use of evidence that the leader can find solutions to the dilemma of standardization versus personalization. Those practices that are known to support safety must be supported, while those practices that are believed to be effective but not supported by evidence can be negotiated.

Evidence indicates that patients who receive care based on the best and latest evidence from well-designed studies experience 28% better outcomes (Heater, Becker, & Olson, 1988). More recent information suggests that in spite of the numerous studies few health-care providers are incorporating research findings into patient care decisions (Melnyk & Fineout-Overholt, 2005).

Leaders can meet the challenge through an intensified focus on first creating the infrastructure and policies that support evidence, then standardization and personalization to assure quality. Evidence-based practice can either integrate the use of published research studies or become the rationale for further study and validation. Integration of a disciplined decision-making process will necessarily support positive outcomes and reduce errors caused from wide variations and personal choice decision making.

Principle #4. Continually Ensure Staff Competence

Effective leadership systems provide the context for the right caregiver doing the right task at the right time, resulting in the right outcome. Leaders serve the system well through creating shared leadership structures in which individuals are accountable for their competence and can identify for the organization when new systems as well as new practices are needed to support technology and research. Quantum leaders serve best by role modeling behaviors of maintaining personal competence and an approach to errors that reflects the philosophy of errors as opportunities. Coupled with the structure, the expectation is that individuals are empowered to risk, to fail, and to be able to optimize personal effectiveness. Lifelong learning in the health-care setting becomes a dynamic process between the leader and accountable professionals.

Strategy: New Approaches for Old Problems

Competence is about more than having knowledge and technical skills; it is also about the physical and mental capacity of the caregiver. Many times, nurses with knowledge and technical skills are exhausted from long hours but continue to work for a variety of reasons, which include both organizational requests and personal needs. Reluctant to let patients down or not meet family commitments, nurses continue to work in highly fatigued states. Given the resounding feedback from nurses and their frustration with excessive patient care assignments and their commitment to the patient, a *claim of conscious* approach may help temper the current adversarial environment.

Nursing is in desperate need of more contemporary vehicles for nurses to objectively express their concerns, discontent, and disillusionments with the work of nursing. The claim of conscience is one strategy that offers a new approach for nurses to address these concerns.

Traditionally, creating claims of conscience clauses has been a strategy to respect practitioner moral and/or religious views. While most conscience clauses require that claims are grounded in religious or moral view, in some jurisdictions claims may be based upon personal judgment or philosophical views.

Claims of conscience components include who is eligible to use the conscience clause, procedures covered by the clause, and principles to be cited when using the clause. In some conscience clauses, the issues are limited to reproductive health or end-of-life issues. The responsibility for evaluating claims of conscience is typically shared across several levels of leadership: the immediate supervisor (attending physician/nurse manager), department chair/director, and administrative executive. Another level includes a review board with members from various ethnic, religious, and academic areas. The review board is intended to represent the diversified demographics within the organization so that all staff might find an advocate.

Creating a new vehicle to address age-old, difficult-to-resolve dilemmas can have a profound application for nursing. The basic principles in evaluating a claim of conscience include:

1. The objection fits within a coherent system of moral, religious, cultural, and philosophical beliefs.
2. This belief reflects a consistently and diligently held core value of the petitioner.
3. The belief is such a key component of the petitioner's internal framework that violation of that belief would cause significant harm to him or her.
4. It would be inconsistent with the petitioner's core values to participate in the procedure or treatment.

Nursing Claims of Conscience

The following is an example of a nursing claim of conscience and serves as a starting point for nurses to discuss complex issues in a framework designed to protect the essence of the discipline of nursing and avoid errors.

1. The objection fits with the nursing code of ethics and is based on a commitment to provide safe, effective, and therapeutic patient care.
2. These beliefs are core beliefs of the nurse. Previous employment records reflect a history of exceptional performance and contributions to the organization and the discipline of nursing.
3. Continued expectations to care for an unreasonable volume and critical level of patients will cause significant stress, probable errors in care, and professional burnout.
4. The nurse is unable to practice under conditions that compromise the core values and beliefs of the profession unless modifications in workload are made.

Attempting to manage the nursing shortage from this perspective creates a new lens from which to examine the work. The outcome must involve negotiation of the workload, prioritization of the specific work to which the nurse is assigned, and elimination of non-value-added, nonurgent work. Mediating the demand for services becomes the approach, rather than continually expecting nurses to assume assignments in which errors are inevitable.

Principle #5. Document Appropriately

The records of the health-care organization provide evidence of services provided, employee history, and the outcomes of those services. Errors in documentation or lack of appropriate documentation can compromise the work of the organization by failing to recognize its essential work, which necessarily includes the documentation of errors.

The leader is accountable for creating systems that identify appropriate documentation and also bears accountability for deliberate falsification or cover-up of information or failure to document care that was given. Finally, assuring timely processes to review the quality of documentation is essential in the creation of a culture of safety. Those doing the documentation must be involved in the review; reviews performed only by external reviewers or quality management specialists decrease the potential for sustainable solutions.

Creating Sustainable Solutions: Engaging Leaders in a Culture of Safety

It is not easy to avoid being too critical, too insensitive, or too demanding in complex cultures when things do go wrong and the past has rendered us victims of the outcomes. One can only hope that tolerance for mistakes will foster innovations and unleash creative solution finding. When leaders are confident that they will not be held to an impossibly high standard, the process of trial and error will enhance the learning process and encourage all individuals to act with the boldness that should be the hallmark of committed healers. Mistakes are not always indicative of future performance. The lessons of the past provide support and guidance to increasing maturity. Resilient leaders absorb the experiences of failure and incorporate them into their ability to evaluate anticipated actions for

---

Leader Documentation Examples

- Strategic plan
- Job descriptions
- Performance evaluations
- Staffing/Scheduling plans and monthly schedules
- Progress summaries
- Service contracts
- Committee records

Quantum Gem

There are not incompetent organizations. Rather, the errors in health care reflect the inherent limits of organizational safety. Recognition of that simple truth is the first and the most important step toward a safer future.

Dr. Kathy A. Scott

the future. In essence, it is the thirst and passion for lifelong learning that drives the leader to reflect honestly on both successes and failures. Further, failures that are not covered up, ignored, or addressed defensively can become the first moment from which lessons can be learned. Much work needs to be done to truly transform the current environment to one that recognizes error as opportunity and expects dialogue among individuals to create a better, more reliable future.

In summary, the following affirmations are offered for the leader aspiring to be effective in managing errors as opportunities.

- I am courageous and consistent in my actions to overcome barriers in achieving the organization's mission.
- My actions and words are consistent even when it would be easier to avoid the issue.
- I expect and encourage discussion of the difficult issues of leadership.
- I do not use my position to fulfill self-interests or further the interests of family, friends, or associates.
- I ensure equitable treatment of patient regardless of socioeconomic group or payor category.
- I demonstrate through organizational policies and discussion with colleagues that overtreatment and undertreatment of patients are unacceptable.
- I protect patients' rights to make their own decisions about care and to have full information about their illnesses, treatment options, and related costs.

REFERENCES

Barnsteiner, J., & Prevost, S. (2002). How to implement evidence-based practice: Some tried and true pointers. *Reflections on Nursing Leadership* 28(2), 18–21.

Benner, P., Sheets, V., Uris, P., Malloch, K., Schwed, K., & Jamison, D. (2002). Individual, practice and system causes of error in nursing. *JONA* 32(10), 509–523.

Chaffee, M. W., & Arthur, D. C. (2002). Failure: Lessons for health care leaders. *Nursing Economic$* 20(5), 225–228, 231.

Cook, R., Render, M., & Woods, D. (2000). Gaps in the continuity of care and progress on patient safety. *British Medical Journal* 320(7237), 791–794.

Deering, A., Dilts, R., & Russell, J. (2003). Leadership cults and cultures. *Leader to Leader* 28, 36–43.

Heater, B., Becker, A., & Olson, R. (1998). Nursing interventions and patient outcomes: A meta-analysis of studies. *Nursing Research* 37, 303–307.

Institute of Medicine. (2001). *Crossing the quality chasm: A new health system for the 21st century.* Washington, DC: National Academy Press.

Kaye, L. (2000). The spiritual roots of mistakes. *The inner edge* 3(2), 5–7.

Leape, L. (1999). The causes and prevention of errors and adverse events in health care. *Image: Journal of Nursing Scholarship* 31(3), 281–286.

Matta, N. F., & Ashkenas, R. N. (2003). Why good projects fail anyway. *Harvard Business Review* 81(9), 109–114.

Melnyk, B. M., & Fineout-Overholt, E. (2005). *Evidence-based practice in nursing and healthcare: A guide to best practice.* Philadelphia, PA: Lippincott, Williams and Wilkins.

Nelson, W. A., & Dark, C. K. (2003). Evaluating claims of conscience. *Healthcare Executive* March–April, 54–55.

Page, A. (Ed.). (2004). *Keeping patients safe: Transforming the work environment of nurses.* Institute of Medicine, Committee on Quality of Health Care in America. Washington, DC: National Academy Press.

Porter-O'Grady, T., & Malloch, K. (2003). *Quantum leadership: A textbook of new leadership.* Sudbury, MA: Jones & Bartlett.

Sagan, S. (1993). *The limits of safety: Organizations, accidents, and nuclear weapons.* Princeton, NJ: Princeton University Press.

Scott, K. A. (2004). Errors and failures in complex health care systems: Individual, team, system and cultural contributors. Unpublished doctoral dissertation, Union Institute & University, Cincinnati, OH.

Ulrich, R., Quan, X., Zimring, C., Joseph, A., & Choudhary, R. (2004, June). *The role of the physical environment in the hospital of the 21st century: A once-in-a-lifetime opportunity.* Preliminary report presented at Designing the 21st Century Hospital Symposium, Washington, DC.

Walshe, K., & Shortell, S. M. (2004). When things go wrong: How health care organizations deal with major failures. *Health Affairs* 23(3), 103–111.

Weick, K., & Sutcliffe, K. (2001). *Managing the unexpected: Assuring high performance in an age of complexity.* San Francisco: Jossey-Bass.

SUGGESTED READING

Hughes, R. G. (2004). First, do no harm: Avoiding near misses. *AJN* 104(5), 81–83.

Rogers, A. E., Hwang, W., Scott, L. D., Aiken, L. H., & Dinges, D. F. (2004). The working hours of hospital staff nurses and patient safety. *Health Affairs* 23(4), 202–212.

Scott, K. A. (2004). Creating highly reliable hospitals through strengthening nursing. *JONA* 34(4), 170–172.

Exercise 1 Scheduling and Safe Staffing

Creating a culture of safety is complex and far-reaching. Given the recent research by Rogers et al. that identifies risk for error after 12 hours of work, identify how your organization will use this evidence.

Examine current schedules for numbers of 12-hour shifts that are associated with overtime.

- How many nurses work more than 40 hours per week?
- What are the error rate/near-miss incidents for this unit?
- Are the majority of errors discussed/reported?
- Request that staff nurses identify what changes need to be made in scheduling practices to control and minimize errors.
- What are the supporting factors and barriers to making changes in scheduling practices and policies?

Exercise 2 Remediate Rather Than Discipline

This chapter has identified five principles to assist the leader in transforming from a culture of error avoidance to a culture that values error as an opportunity to create a better future that includes improving processes.

In a small group discuss each principle and do the following:

- Identify the level of performance/competence for each principle as an individual and as a team.
- Develop a plan to celebrate and share the competency achievements with others in the organization.
- Identify actions that would improve leader behaviors.
- Prioritize the actions and develop a plan to achieve greater error management competency as individuals and as a team.

Transforming Leader Behaviors	Errors to Avoid
1. Know yourself	• Lack of self-awareness of skills and impact on the environment/colleagues • Lack of engagement and presence with the health-care system • Interpreting the present in terms of past successes • Failure to inspire and create a powerful guiding coalition • Undercommunicating the vision
2. Plan for error	• Lack of attentiveness • Failing to develop new ways of filtering and managing information; processing information through old perspectives • Supporting/tolerating complacency • Overreliance on memory • Retaining unnecessary procedures • Failure to assure safe work schedules • Failure to assure safe physical environment
3. Balance standardization and personalization	• Lack of or faulty intervention due to lack of information; lack of skill • Continuation of overly complex and confusing processes • Overcontrolling information access • Egotistical invincibility—my way is best!
4. Continually assure staff competence	• Lack of advocacy/professional responsibility • Failing to create short-term wins • Lack of passion for the work of nursing • Assigning unprepared staff to perform complex tasks
5. Documentation	• Inaccurate documentation • Failure to document essential activities of patients, caregivers, and the system

Victim Statements

The following statements are common victim statements. As you read each statement, ask yourself "Does this apply to me?" or "Have I ever felt this way?" Validate your assessments with a colleague. Develop strategies to minimize *victimness* as a means to creating a culture that views error as opportunity rather than one looking to pinpoint blame.

1. I have been surprised by negative feedback from someone when I thought all along I was doing my very best to solve a problem.
2. I have spent time blaming others and pointing fingers when things did not go the way I wanted them to go.
3. I have spent time "covering my tail" (sending cc: or bcc: e-mail messages) just in case things went wrong.
4. In the last month, I have said, "It's not my job" and expected someone else to solve a problem.
5. At least once a week, I have felt totally powerless, with no control over my circumstances or situation.
6. At times, I have found myself "waiting to see if" a situation would miraculously resolve itself.
7. At times, I am so frustrated that I have said, "Just tell me what you want me to do and I'll do it."

CHAPTER 6

The Fully Engaged Leader

CHAPTER OBJECTIVES:

Upon completion of this chapter, the reader will:

1. Understand the attributes of the fully engaged leader and the relationships of engagement to organizational outcomes.
2. Review the theoretical underpinnings of the emotional aspects of leadership and the challenges of integrating these concepts into leadership development.
3. Discuss the significance of the leadership calling as an integral component of engagement.
4. Appreciate three processes of engagement skill building: self-assessment, valuing others, and sustaining engagement.

INTRODUCTION

An estimated 40% of all managers fail in the first 18 months on the job (Carnes, Cottrell & Layton, 2004). The costs to the organization and to individuals are significant and beg for approaches that will improve the success rate. Unfortunately, the attributes separating successful managers from those who fail are often elusive. No cookie-cutter recipe for leader success has been identified despite numerous studies by leadership experts.

Leader success depends on a wide range of variables that are related to the work to be done, the skills and abilities of the leader and the team, the needs of the team members, the resources available, and the motivation of all those involved. To be sure, this list is not inclusive and it continually evolves. The *right stuff* of leadership may indeed have common characteristics and behaviors, but the reality is that each leader has a unique combination of multiple characteristics, values, behaviors, and ability to get the work done. Most leaders develop their personal essence on the basis of education, experience, mental intelligence, emotional intelligence, and the ability to form meaningful relationships.

This chapter presents the emerging profile of the engaged leader to gain a greater appreciation of the complexity of leadership and the sig-

Key Concepts

Consciousness

Awareness of one's own existence, sensations, thoughts, surroundings; the thoughts and feelings, collectively, of an individual or of an aggregate of people.

Competence

The quality of having suitable or sufficient skill, knowledge, and experience for some purpose; properly qualified.

Intelligence

Capacity for learning, reasoning, and understanding; aptitude in grasping truths, relationships, facts, meanings; mental alertness or quickness of understanding.

Engagement

The act of being involved or committed to something; a pledge, an obligation or an agreement.

Ten Principles of Complexity

1. Wholes are made up of parts.
2. All health care is local.
3. Adding value to a part adds value to the whole.
4. Simple systems make up complex systems.
5. Diversity is a necessity of life.
6. Error is essential to creation.
7. Systems thrive when all of their functions intersect and interact.
8. Equilibrium and disequilibrium are in constant tension.
9. Change is generated from the center outward.
10. Revolution results from the aggregation of local changes.

Porter-O'Grady & Malloch, 2003

Self-Reflection: Observe Yourself

Body Language

- Eye contact, arms folded/unfolded

Timing of responses

- Quick, slow, not at all

Inclusion/exclusion of others in discussions

Ask your colleagues to share feedback about your body language, timeliness, and inclusion practices. Is it consistent with your assessment? Which behaviors should be retained? Changed?

nificance of engagement as a leader characteristic, and to stimulate discussion of the potential impact of engaged behaviors on organizational performance. A brief review of the emotional intelligence literature, processes of the development of engagement, and a new employee interview template that integrates the notions of engagement within a culture of transformation are also presented.

The engaged leader in a health-care organization has highly developed technical and emotional competence and is fully focused on the work to be done, the necessary relationships to get the work done, and the ever-changing mood of the organization. The environment created by the emotionally competent leader supports employees to experience their own emotions, set limits on expressions when appropriate, and encourages others to be similarly empowered.

First and foremost, emotionally competent leaders acknowledge and respect their own feelings and have the awareness and discipline to not be distracted by the anxieties and stresses of the moment; they actively direct their emotional energy into doing the right thing in the right way, at the right time. Emotionally competent leaders not only make self-awareness a priority and are unafraid of their feelings but also work to understand the impact they have on others. This high level of consciousness about personal impact is foundational for leaders who are fully engaged in the work of health care, with colleagues and the organization, and, finally, to continuing personal growth. To be sure, it is no small feat to become a fully engaged leader.

Necessarily, the leader with a high level of emotional competence is not at an end point. Rather, the leader is positioned to continually transcend to higher levels of consciousness, using the skills of emotional competence to relate with others in ways that were previously not possible.

COMPLEXITY LIVE!

Emotionally competent leaders do not dispute or debate the interrelatedness of the processes of leadership, which includes the technical skills of leadership, intentionality, and emotional competence. Perhaps there is no better portrayal of the notion of complexity than what is found in fully engaged leaders and the relationships they form as the means to transform work and the workplace, help others own their own change, undertake the right change processes, and integrate the rules of engagement for the postindustrial age. Engaged leaders are able to both act and reflect upon the events and processes of leading that emphasize the short term but integrate the long-term needs of the community. The complex nature of all health care relationships reflects the inescapable interrelationships of all things in the world and the ten principles of complexity (Porter-O'Grady & Malloch, 2003).

Rather than being overwhelmed by the complex nature of work to be done, the pace of change, the limitations of time, and the endless advances in technology, the fully engaged leader thrives within the following realities of complexity theory:

- Change is endless
- Information is more readily available than ever
- Knowledge is no longer a possession but rather an access or utility for good leadership
- Technology changes the character and content of the health-care service relationship

Becoming competent in the technical skills of leadership and creating clear organizational goals is much less challenging than developing expertise in building and maintaining relationships, which reflects a high level of emotional competence. Mastery of these *people skills* is a basic expectation for all leaders, yet the attainment of expertise in relationship-building skills continues to challenge even the most experienced health-care leaders. As leaders gain an appreciation of the principles of complexity theory and integrate the ideas into the work of leadership, the challenges of new relationships, new technology, and new regulations become much more manageable. Thus, the engaged leader with expertise in technical leadership and relationship building has identified her or his personal and professional purposes and vision for the future and is able to actively facilitate the transformational processes for others. The realties of complexity for the engaged leader include:

- The undeniable interrelationships between all individuals in the organization and the community
- An emphasis on local health care, namely, the work that occurs at the point of care between the patient and the caregiver
- Multiple perspectives as essential for survival
- Failure as an opportunity for improvement
- CHANGE just IS!

In spite of the undeniable reality of these challenges, commitment to the journey that requires leaders to be emotionally competent and fully engaged is not always valued. Significant pressures emphasize the technical work of strategic planning, budgeting, and controlling. Time and energy to develop relationships or the soft side of leadership are viewed as luxuries, given that they are not believed to be necessarily related to the net income margin.

Developing the people skills of leadership—regardless of what label or attribute is attached to them—provides the most effective vehicle for sustained learning to occur through the recognized power of the collective emotions of the team. It is through people's full engagement with their work that the measurable, sustainable results of satisfaction, quality outcomes, and strong net income margins are achieved. Organizations continue to struggle not only to recognize the quantifiable value of emotional competence but also to inexorably link these attributes to technical leadership processes. Continual reinforcement and demonstration of these relationships is a never-ending process for engaged and enlightened leaders.

UNDERSTANDING THE PAST: FOUNDATIONS FOR ENGAGEMENT

The evolving body of knowledge dedicated to understanding and guiding people in developing an engaged leadership competence that integrates technical and relational skills continues to offer new and differing perspectives for the leader. Much has been written about the ways in which individuals deal with their emotions, emotions that are an integral part of every leader's personal essence. It is through the understanding of the nature and dynamics of emotions that leaders are able to advance in their journey to a state of full engagement.

Recent variations in the descriptions of emotional intelligence (EI) have raised concerns for some scholars. Some also believe that the significance of EI has been overstated due to the lack of evidence supporting the relationship between emotional intelligence and workplace success (Vitello-Cicciu, 2002). In spite of the criticisms of the lack of conceptual clarity and overriding behaviors, the basic notions of this work continue to

---

Emotionally Competent Behaviors

- Soliciting opinions of team members in meetings
- Listening until the other person is finished talking
- Able to deal with disappointment

Emotionally Incompetent Behaviors

- Yelling at another person
- Rejecting or dismissing the opinions and ideas of others
- Gossip
- Whirlwinds of hyperactivity
- Distraught over disappointments

The Teddy Bear Factor

Emotional Intelligence involves more than being introspective. It also involves what I call the Teddy Bear Factor—do people feel comfortable with you? Do they want to be close to you?

Manfred F.R. Kets de Vries

Goleman's 25 EI Competencies (1998)

1. Emotional awareness
2. Accurate self-assessment
3. Self-confidence
4. Self-control
5. Trustworthiness
6. Conscientiousness
7. Adaptability
8. Innovation
9. Achievement drive
10. Commitment
11. Initiative
12. Optimism
13. Understanding others
14. Developing others
15. Service orientation
16. Leveraging diversity
17. Political awareness
18. Influence
19. Communication
20. Conflict management
21. Leadership
22. Change catalyst
23. Building bonds
24. Collaboration
25. Team capabilities

Gem

The way a question is asked limits and disposes the ways in which any answer to it—right or wrong—may be given.

Susanne K. Langer

Gem

Soulful leaders are containers for the "ands" and work diligently to eliminate the "either and or's."

enlighten many leaders about the complexities of emotions and their impact on the workplace.

Given that the theoretical underpinnings of emotional intelligence reflect theories of emotion, motivation, behavior, intelligence, organizational behavior, and neuroscience, its complexity is readily apparent. The intersections and overlapping of one's feelings, sense of purpose, knowledge, and attitude vary widely and often unpredictably. New perspectives and new approaches to further engagement and expertise in relationship building can still be learned from the study of the emotional intelligence literature.

The concept of emotional intelligence is significant to understanding emotions. The early definers of EI, Slaovey and Mayer (Vitello-Cicciu, 2002), identified three processes as its essence: appraisal and expression of emotion, regulation of emotion, and utilization of emotion. Further studies extended this understanding of EI from one of personal assessment to one that includes the understanding of the emotions of others. New theories identified the ability to perceive emotions, to access and/or generate feeling to assist one's thoughts, and to understand emotional knowledge. Given that the predominant assumption regarding EI is that emotions and intelligence are connected, not all theorists interpreted EI as consistent with the notion of intelligence. Some have misinterpreted the notion of intelligence beyond the definition of mental performance to personality traits, thus creating conceptual confusion (Vitello-Cicciu, 2002).

Goleman (1995) followed the work of Salovey and Mayer and defined emotional intelligence as "the ability to motivate oneself and persist in the face of frustration; to control impulses and delay gratification; to regulate one's moods and keep distress from swamping the ability to think; to emphasize and to hope" (p. 34). The five broad categories of EI defined by Goleman (1995) are: self-awareness, self-regulation, motivation, empathy, and social skills. These are more aligned with motivational intelligence than with EI (Vitello-Cicciu, 2002). Twenty-five competencies have been further identified by Goleman (1998).

These complex phenomena within emotional intelligence are difficult to discretely compartmentalize, and thus they further challenge leadership development experts. While some believe it is difficult for leaders to develop specific standardized approaches to facilitating high levels of emotional competence, the many supporting theories do indeed offer differing areas of focus for leadership development.

Given the recent emphasis on emotional intelligence or the *soft side* of leadership, leaders have struggled to avoid artificial labels and artificial goals that are based solely on the emotional intelligence aspect and thereby fragment the essence of the integrated leadership perspective. Some leaders have identified values, preferred behaviors, and decision-making styles through the Myers-Briggs Inventory, the DISC-Performax assessment, and numerous other assessment tools in addition to the EI survey, gaining an understanding of not only emotional skills but also interpersonal decision-making skills.

At times leaders become overfocused on the style and behaviors of leadership to the extent where one's style (Myers-Briggs or DISC) is identified on the employee badge. Both leaders and employees become focused on the style of decision making at the expense of the desired outcomes. While it is certainly relevant to know that some individuals may be an *ENTJ* and make decisions more quickly than others, this information is one piece of the data and does not take into consideration the current context of events and interactions. When there is a need to respond quickly to assure patient safety, the end goal of patient safety must be primary, while individual styles are secondary or in some situations irrelevant. The fact that one's primary behavior or decision-making style reflects the need for time to process is secondary to the contextual realities of the situation. The fully engaged leader assures focus on the desired, value-based outcomes that support quality patient care service while information specific to style is supportive but not the driver of processes.

Many scholars continue to offer guidelines for leadership, but there is no widely accepted standardized template of behaviors for effective leadership. Outcomes of good leadership have been identified more consistently than behaviors such as the achievement of clinical outcomes, employee satisfaction, and fiscal stability, which integrate and reflect the unique values, beliefs, and skills of the organization. Regardless of the approach or theoretical underpinning selected by the leader to guide the development of interpersonal or soft skills, the process of development must always be directed to the outcomes; processes must never overtake the significance of the desired outcomes. As previously noted, working to identify one's decision-making style and focusing on the need for expression of that style in deference to achieving organizational goals is inappropriate. The goal is to understand one's style and integrate it into the group decision-making process and achieve the desired goal.

Three developmental processes are identified to assist leaders along the pathway of engagement. The first is discovering the authentic you, the second is valuing others, and the third is sustaining the essence of engagement. Each of these processes is presented with strategies and values that are designed to assist you along your journey.

THE AUTHENTIC SELF: A CALLING OF LEADERSHIP

Some days the work of leadership seems like more than a person can handle, yet dedicated leaders continue on through seemingly insurmountable challenges. Most likely, the work of leadership has become an internal calling. The calling to leadership or the inner urge to give away one's gifts and make distinct contributions to the world not only uncovers the joy that everyone seeks but also affirms one's life work and contributions to a better world. It is the calling to leadership that energizes, affirms, and sustains leaders in times of great challenge.

According to Leider (2004), engaged leaders not only know who they are and what they stand for but also are able to assist others to heed their own life callings. They are able to guide others to uncover their embedded destiny and to see beyond today to what they can become tomorrow. This is the ultimate coaching and mentoring process! Thus, the engaged leader with emotional competence is able both to identify personal destiny and to assist others in the journey of discovery and commitment to their calling as a part of the larger design of the world. Not surprising, engaged leaders recognize their calling not as a destiny or goal, but as a wellness issue; leading is doing what needs to be done, and not doing the work of leadership would be frustrating and stress producing.

The calling of leadership guides the leader in integrating the internal personal self with the outer world, a struggle that is continuously present in many leaders. Knowing from the internal self what needs to be done and living those beliefs and values in the real world marks the leader's journey. The leader must role model the integration of the personal, authentic self with the real, external world. The journey starts with the self and moves toward others and the needs of the world. The fully engaged leader emulates a high level of consciousness or spiritual connection with

> ### Gem
>
> Information voids will be filled by rumors and speculation unless they are preempted by open, credible and trustworthy communication. Pull no punches. When you know an answer, give it. When you don't, say so. When you're guessing, admit it. But don't stop communication.
>
> Jean B. Keffeler

> ### The Calling of Leadership
>
> Humans search for meaning. Life has some meaning because there is some good in it. The most meaningful lives are the ones in which we directly serve others. Calling joins self and service. When our talents and the needs of the world cross, there lies our vocation.
>
> Richard Leider, 2004

those in the world. The leader is fully present in each situation, listens carefully with an open mind, and, on the basis of core values, interacts assertively and honestly.

THE AUTHENTIC SELF: INTEGRITY

As noted previously, an essential quality that the engaged leader must have is to be his or her own person, to be authentic in every way. Any prospective leader who buys into the necessity of copying the characteristics of other leaders is doomed to fail. Those who are too responsive to others, too quick to deviate from the plan, or unwilling to make difficult decisions for fear of offending others are likely to be overridden by competitors, either internal or external. The authentic leader works to know and be him- or herself.

Within every leader are the questions: What is my professional identity? What do I stand for? Examples of areas of self-awareness that the engaged leader examines include the very basic:

- What is important to me? Balance, family, work, success?
- Do I value stability, innovation, wealth, happiness, humor?
- What makes me happy, sad, laugh, cry, stressed, calm?
- Are behaviors that are gregarious, energetic, impulsive, quiet, shy tolerable to me?
- How do I treat others? With respect, indifference, selectively?
- What impact do I want to have on others? To be liked, loved, respected?
- How do I react to failure? To myself, to others who fail?
- How do I describe myself? How do others describe me?

Engaged leaders focus on the deepest dimension of that which defines their uniqueness and potential: the authentic self. Leaders with high degrees of awareness of themselves and those in their environment are described as not just engaged or sensitive to the activities between two people, but sensitive to the larger environment, to the location, other individuals, and the ramifications of the endless interrelationships of the world at large. Consciousness of not only their own self but also the impact of the presence of others and the interactions in which they are involved is a way of being for soulful, engaged leaders. They are known for their continual work in increasing self-understanding of their strengths, weaknesses, values, beliefs, and passions and are able to demonstrate ownership of their behaviors, both the behaviors that contribute positively to harmony and behaviors that are less than perfect. Self-knowledge is achieved in many ways through a lifelong commitment to examination of values, behaviors, accomplishments, and most importantly, the impact on others.

THE AUTHENTIC SELF: NARCISSISTIC

Although it may be difficult for some leaders to acknowledge, narcissism is an essential leadership trait. According to Kets de Vries (Coutu, 2004), all people need a healthy dose of narcissism in order to survive, especially leaders. Narcissism is the engine that drives leadership; assertiveness, self-confidence, tenacity, and creativity are essential to lead. The challenge is to not go over the edge and adopt autocratic behaviors, thus destroying shared decision-making processes. Indeed, leaders can be quite successful in facilitating team processes as assertive, confident, tenacious, and creative individuals. The challenge for leaders is to not overwhelm team members so they become a mirror image of the leader, idealizing and uncritically accepting whatever the leader proposes.

Quantum Gem

The leader's first job is to define reality.

The last is to say thank you.

In between the leader must become a servant and a debtor.

Max DePree,
Former Chairman Herman Miller

Quantum Gem

How can we communicate love? I think three things are involved:

We must reach out to a person, make contact.

We must listen with the heart, be sensitive to the other's needs.

We must respond in a language that the person can understand. Many of us do all the talking. We must learn to listen and to keep on listening.

Princess Pale Moon

Quantum Gem

Dimensions of Authentic Leaders

1. Understanding their purpose
2. Practicing solid values
3. Leading with heart
4. Demonstrating self-discipline

Bill George, 2004

THE AUTHENTIC SELF:
TRUTH TELLER—THE WHOLE TRUTH,
HALF OF THE TRUTH, OR MY LIPS ARE SEALED?

Authentic leaders behave consistently with identified values and beliefs that have been developed through reflection, study, and dialogue with others. These values form the leader's moral compass. There is a deep sense of what is right and what is wrong. Further, authentic leaders value integrity, which is not just the absence of lying but is telling the whole truth, no matter how painful it might be. Sharing of partial information may be less painful, but sharing of all information is expected by the authentic leader. Telling the whole truth is natural to the authentic leader, just as is admitting mistakes when one falls short and does not succeed. This demonstrates courage to be authentic and honest in all situations.

Engaged leaders speak the truth in a caring, compassionate way, even when the news is not pleasant. Authenticity requires courage to respond when it is easier to be silent and noncommittal and requires courage to avoid partial truths. The lack of response implies agreement to most observers, an impression engaged leaders do not want to give.

Authenticity also often involves telling the stories that no one else will tell, stories that reflect the essence of the human spirit and feelings that range from despair to anger to disappointment. One example involves the termination of a "favored" employee by a new leader. After finding significant performance issues, the new leader documented the behaviors and began termination procedures. When the new leader informed her supervisor, who previously had been the employee's supervisor, of her decision to terminate, the response from the supervisor was less than typical, but very authentic. The previous supervisor first provided her support to the new leader and then noted that the problem behavior had indeed been present for some time and that she had failed to address it. She thanked the new leader for her integrity and willingness to address a significant issue, something she had been unable to do for a variety of reasons such as a long history with the employee, other priorities, and concern that she would not be able to follow through completely. The sharing of these stories serves many purposes: building relationships, understanding human frailty, and the willingness to recognize that at times others can do a more effective job that you yourself are able to do. Some may perceive this as a failure of leadership rather than the reality of life steeped in complexity, uncertainty, and trial and error. Certain events result from particular combinations of context, timing, and personal energy, rather than behaviors that reflect poor leadership.

Finally, the authentic, engaged leader avoids the tendency to "depersonalize" a situation, to blame it on an objective entity such as "the system." The authentic, fully engaged leader recognizes that individuals create the organization and its culture and are thus the only ones able to change or improve it. Rarely does the leader hide behind the shield of system policies; rather, the leader owns the system policies and is accountable to examine and modify policies if the outcomes can be improved.

Discussion

Authenticity is recognized through both obvious truthfulness and subtle messages. Consider the following three questions.

1. Is there such a thing as a truthful budget? Why do some organizations expect an absolute budget that is only negotiated once a year?
   Why do some believe that the budgeting process is used as a shield to discourage some expenditures and at other times to provide flexibility for an uncertain future? Why do some leaders believe the budget is a guideline rather than an absolute and specific allocation of resources?
2. Is the performance appraisal ever totally honest?
   Or is the process a reflection of partial, nonspecific information that minimizes the opportunity for healthy dialogue and ultimately employee growth?
3. Which principle(s) of complexity guide each perspective?

When wealth is lost, nothing is lost;

When health is lost, something is lost;

When character is lost, all is lost.

                                    German proverb

VALUING OTHERS:
LISTENING FROM THE HEART

There can never be enough emphasis on listening to others with a stilled mind. Soulful leaders use a communication style that begins with personal focus and clearing of the mind, questions for greater understanding, and then response. Receptive, open communication is about the willingness to embrace many perspectives and creative ideas.

Quantum Gem

The real art of conversation is not to say the right thing in the right place but to leave unsaid the wrong thing at the tempting moment.

Lady Dorothy Nevill

Avoiding a Hall of Mirrors

1. Focus on vision and values
2. Make sure people disagree
3. Cultivate truth tellers
4. Do as you would have done to you
5. Honor your intuition
6. Delegate, don't desert

Offerman, 2004

Finding Common Ground

Adversaries are often believed to be arch-enemies; yet, there can be common ground that once identified can be used to mediate the conflict-ridden situation. Consider the following four relationships that are often adversarial:

- Physician — Nurse
- Labor union — Professional practice advocates
- Day shift — Night shift
- Finance — Nursing

Identify three specific areas of common ground for each of the dyads of conflict.

Identify three specific areas of conflict for each of the dyads of conflict.

Can you identify new ways to create new and better relationships within the dyads?

The engaged leader not only recognizes that there are many perspectives within a team or organization but also seeks out the differing viewpoints in order to recognize and give value to all dimensions. Efforts are not focused on eliminating the differing ideas but rather on working to sustain healthy tensions in which diverse polarities are present: peace and war, conservative and liberal, nursing and non-nursing, traditional medicine and alternative therapies. There is no rubber stamping of like-minded ideas or like-minded individuals.

Receptive communicators also understand the importance of "suffering presence," which is the willingness to tolerate (while perhaps suffering on the inside) others' viewpoints, values, beliefs, thinking styles, and even the same story for the second time. Receptive communicators are truly present; they are engaged in the dialogue and are not merely marking time until they can interrupt and speak their mind. Finally, receptive communicators do not intimidate others in order to make a point or gain support for their position.

VALUING OTHERS: AVOIDING THE RUBBER STAMP

The established, successful leader can be unintentionally intimidating to others, particularly new members of the team. Engaged leaders do not want members of the team to merely echo their ideas and proposals, even when they are new to the team. Engaged leaders create the context for open, healthy dialogue to elicit new ideas, discard suboptimal processes, and create new strategies from the collective wisdom of the team.

Resisting the power of flattery is an important skill that is seldom taught in management programs. The quantum leader is well served to periodically examine the dynamics of the team and affirm that he or she is not in a hall of mirrors, being continually flattered and reinforced, hearing only ideas that echo those of the leader, and seldom receiving challenging feedback. The leader does not need mirror images of him- or herself; it is healthy debate and dialogue that is needed by the leader to achieve great results.

Engaged leaders are sensitive to the tendency to quash creativity, and they work to avoid responses such as, "We've always done it this way" or "We tried that last year and it didn't work." Continuing emphasis is placed on eliminating these reactions from both the leader's and other members' vocabularies.

VALUING OTHERS: FINDING COMMON GROUND

Finding common ground when it seems nonexistent is also a characteristic behavior of the engaged leader. Rather than allow conflicts to persist, leaders brainstorm with those who may have differing ideas and work to identify areas of common interest that can be used to reinstate healthy dialogue and minimize conflict. Too often, the emphasis is on differences rather than on finding areas of common ground that could serve to begin healthy dialogue. Negative issues may be highlighted rather than mediated. For each conflicting situation, there is always common ground to be identified. It may begin with the commonality of being a health-care worker, the need for a job, or the current shift worked. Other commonalities that can serve as openings for less stressful conversations include gender, age group, ethnic background, birthplace, college attended, and sports interests. Once dialogue has begun in a less stressful manner, individuals can move on to discussing and resolving areas of conflict.

VALUING OTHERS: ENDURING RELATIONSHIPS

The capacity to develop close and enduring relationships is one mark of a leader. The detached style of leadership in which leaders remain aloof from those they supervise does not work in today's workplace. Employees demand more personal relationships with their leaders before they will give themselves fully to their job (George, 2004). They expect access to leaders and know that openness and the depth of relationships with the leader are the foundations for trust and commitment to the organization. These enduring relationships—the soft skill outcome—are built on connectedness and shared purposes and serve as an important element in achieving far-reaching and once believed impossible goals.

> ### Self-Awareness: My Legacy
>
> As a leader, the legacy you leave can range from a very positive difference, no perceived change, or a very negative impact.
>
> Consider your legacy on a daily basis:
>
> What difference did you make today?
>
> Who did you affect?
>
> What opportunities did you miss?
>
> What do you need to change?

VALUING OTHERS: COMPETING FAIRLY

Leaders are highly competitive individuals driven to succeed in whatever they take on. Authentic leaders know that competing requires self-discipline in order to be successful. There are two views of competition: the positive or win-win side and a negative or win-lose side. When individuals compete with each other to establish superior and subordinate positions, namely, someone wins and someone loses, competition is considered negative. When individuals compete against their own performance to achieve higher levels, the competition takes on a more positive aspect. There are only winners in this approach; the past is improved upon, and new outcomes increase the value of the results. For example, when patient care units compete against each other for the highest patient satisfaction scores, one unit always wins and the others lose. It is seldom possible for an oncology unit to exceed the satisfaction scores of a postpartum unit due to the nature of the clinical situation. It is possible for each unit to compete with last month's score and work to achieve higher ratings within the unit. All units can potentially be winners.

Being competitive does not have to be negative; it is an essential quality of successful leaders, but it needs to be channeled through purpose and discipline. It is not uncommon to mistake competitive individuals, those who generate results by improving organizational effectiveness, for genuine leaders. Achieving operational effectiveness is an essential result for any leader, but it alone does not ensure authenticity or long-term success.

SUSTAINING ENGAGEMENT: SELF-DEVELOPMENT

To be sure, the need for a lifetime learning process requires discipline, but it is the internal passion to want to learn more about new ideas, historical perspectives, and the successes or failures of initiatives that creates sustainable learning. Yet, sometimes having passion for learning is not enough in the complex and ever-changing health-care environment. Much has been written about the importance of continuing development and lifelong learning for both individuals and organizations as the vehicle to continually examine processes and reinvent the workplace to sustain marketplace competitiveness. The imbalance of excessive operational demands often displaces the preferred balance that integrates operations, continuing development, and time and energy management, further challenging the engaged leader to determine effective strategies to regain the balance.

According to Edgar Schein (Coutu, 2002), in reality few companies ever succeed in genuinely reinventing themselves; they rarely get to the point of challenging deeply held assumptions about strategies and processes

Discussion

Coercive Persuasion and the EMR

Edgar Schein, noted organizational theorist, described *coercive persuasion* as a situation in which people cannot physically escape and are pressured into adopting new beliefs.

Consider the emergence of the electronic medical record (EMR) and its impact on caregiver behavior and the use of paper. Giving up or at least minimizing the printing of reports and using notebooks in favor of the electronic devices is a significant challenge for all caregivers.

Removing printers and the supply of paper is an example of coercive persuasion. What other examples have occurred in your organization?

Do you agree that change or learning occurs best through coercive persuasion? Why? Why not?

and thinking and acting in fundamentally altered ways. Rather, most end up doing the same thing in superficially tweaked ways—practices that fall short of what is needed to compete in the 21st century. Further, Schein (Coutu, 2002) notes that in spite of the optimistic rhetoric that learning is fun, learning is often more about guilt and anxiety. Indeed some may enjoy and revel in the learning process, but more change is believed to be accomplished through indoctrination and coercive persuasion!

Engaged leaders are indeed accountable for their own lifelong learning. They are sensitive to the radical ideas of coercive persuasion and realize that there is an inherent paradox surrounding learning; anxiety inhibits learning, but anxiety is also necessary if learning is going to occur. For many, the presence of anxiety stimulates and reinforces the need for change, given that real change begins after the organization or the individual experiences some threat that thwarts progress or desired outcomes. The leader works with the anxiety of learning and channels activities into situations in which people learn together, minimizing the anxiety of looking foolish in the process.

Consider the recent organizational changes to support patient safety initiatives. Patient safety has always been important to health-care workers, in spite of the documented high numbers of errors and tweaking of the systems that resulted in errors. Not until major reports from the Institute of Medicine were presented did significant change in practices specific to patient safety begin—an example of coercive persuasion. Organizations were mandated by regulatory and accrediting agencies to make specific changes within defined time frames. Such learning and change is indeed reality, and the engaged leader works to use both the anxiety of the situation and the dedication of health-care workers to create sustainable solutions that improve patient safety outcomes.

SUSTAINING ENGAGEMENT: MEASURING SUCCESS

The measuring stick of the highly engaged leader is more than the accumulation of wealth, jewelry, homes, and automobiles. The engaged leader perceives success as much more than material goods. Enduring success is the result of multiple forces and multiple skills: success gets leaders where they want to be, with rewards that are sustainable for them and those they care about. It is about success that is emotionally renewing, not anxiety provoking.

Further, each engaged leader perceives and values success in unique ways that may indeed change over time. There is no standardized format for success; rather there are commonalities that serve to nourish the mind, body, and spirit. Nash and Stevenson (2004) identified four components of enduring success:

Discussion

Enduring Success

Nash and Stevenson (2004) have identified four components for enduring success: happiness, achievement, significance, and legacy. In a group, consider each of the four components and identify as many possible examples of each component that are unique to nurses.

Which area of success is the easiest to attain?

Which one(s) are the most challenging?

How can you develop a more balanced approach to achieving enduring success?

Who can assist you along the way?

- Happiness: feelings of pleasure or contentment about one's life
- Achievement: accomplishments that compare favorably against similar goals others have strived for
- Significance: the sense that one has made a positive impact on people one cares about
- Legacy: the way to establish one's values or accomplishments so as to help others find future success

Each of these components is important in creating feelings of success. For example, achieving significant wealth from a corporate position without the ability to experience pleasure does not lend to a feeling of success. Or, if one had a significant power base of thousands of employees but did not allow for the creation of positive impacts on others, success would also not be felt. Success is never satisfied by just one category; it encompasses one's personal life, achievement at work, significance to family, and legacy to the community.

Engaged health-care leaders recognize the need for balance and focus in all four categories; focusing on one factor leads to knowing that you are doing what is right but still feeling unsuccessful. The achievements and pleasure of one category fade as soon as they occur. Working diligently to create a legacy without sensitivity to operational responsibilities, failing to spend time with family, and unhealthy diet and exercise habits become short-lived and frustrating.

In contrast, enduring success that recognizes all four categories is enriching and sustainable. Synergy is created in single events and the combination of activities. As the leader takes time for family and coworkers while creating a new health-care center, giving to the community, and attending continuing education workshops, the balance of activities is focused and sustainable. The integration of activities at this level does not occur without thought and reflection and regular adjustments.

SUSTAINING ENGAGEMENT: SOULFUL OPTIMISM

Engaged leaders are filled with optimism and resilience, filled with belief that the future is brighter and that one can indeed make a difference. They understand that disharmony or stress is caused by forces external to them in the world and that the way to reduce stress is to gain internal control, not more control of the world. For example, when the engaged leader is caught in a traffic jam, the stress level does not automatically increase due the annoyance of being late; rather, the slowdown is managed as an opportunity to relax. The challenge is to change the view of the world from the inside to sustain calm and harmony!

HIRING FOR ENGAGEMENT AND PRESENCE: THE BANNER ESTRELLA MODEL

Interviewing for and retaining employees who are committed to full engagement in the organizational culture begins with an interviewing process that is aligned with organizational values among all employees, not just those in leadership positions. As a new facility, Banner Estrella Medical Center (BEMC) recognized the incredible opportunity to create the ultimate organizational culture and physical environment supportive of healing and at the same time to remedy behaviors that had been barriers to quality patient outcomes, a safe environment, and employee satisfaction. BEMC leaders worked with the community to identify the desired values, services, and outcomes that would support the best health care possible. The collective effort not only identified the characteristics of the physical facility that would architecturally support healing, but also the culture that would transform the health-care experience.

Early in the process, the newly hired leadership team created an interviewing template that integrated core values and behaviors of the parent organization, Banner Health, and the expectations for all employees seeking to be a part of the transformational culture. The team clearly appreciated this opportunity to correct previous undesirable behaviors and practices and thus created an interview template to guide all interviewers and interviewees in identifying and selecting employees with consistent values and motivation to participate in the transformation. The interviewing template follows at the end of the chapter in Appendix 1.

SUMMARY

Achieving full engagement is not a destination; it is a lifetime journey that is filled with varying degrees of engagement. Leaders may be focused and fully engaged in the work at hand. Or leaders may be overchallenged by the intensity and quantity of work, personal health status, and family needs, and are thus unable to be engaged at the desired level. Recognizing the difference and accepting the reality is healthy and stress reducing for the engaged, emotionally competent leader. Achieving full engagement in a world based on complexity theory is at best a highly sought-after state that exists only intermittently, based on the degree of change present in the modern world, available time, and technological advances. Continuing activity limits the opportunity for minor engagement with others and the system, much less full engagement. This is not to dissuade leaders from striving for engagement as means to improve relationship effectiveness and outcomes, but it is a reminder of the reality of a world steeped in complexity.

It is much like reaching for the stars; the destination is ever present and inspirational. The lack of success in reaching a star does not deter one from continuing to envision the process and continually aspire to greater achievements.

Exercise 1 Discovering Full Engagement

The profile of the fully engaged leader includes the following characteristics:

- A high level of self-awareness with specific criteria that have emerged over time
- Valuing others
- Commitment to continuing development
- Application of values and beliefs to daily operations

For each of the four characteristics, list the behaviors and specific actions that should be taken to assure a high level of engagement. Also, identify behaviors that should be eliminated to improve engagement.

Exercise 2 The Hall of Mirrors

Healthy dialogue requires sharing opinions, challenging assumptions, and encouraging new ideas. Leaders may find themselves in a hall of mirrors, with everyone agreeing and praising the leader for his or her views, proposals, and progress. No one challenges the leader. Often the result is organizational dysfunction, a disrespectful culture, and little or no progress.

Are you in a hall of mirrors?

Consider proposing an unrealistic idea and assess the response. If the response is the mirror of yourself, begin to assess the behaviors and rational, for member reluctance to engage in healthy dialogue.

Identify at least one strategy to support open dialogue and decrease the rubber stamping of ideas.

Identify the potential improvements as a result of this change.

REFERENCES

Carnes, K., Cottrell, D., & Layton, M. C. (2004). *Management insights: Discovering the truths to management success*. Dallas, TX: CornerStone Leadership Institute.

Coutu, D. L. (2004). Putting leaders on the couch: A conversation with Manfred F. R. Kets de Vries. *Harvard Business Review* 82(1), 65–71.

Coutu, D. L. (2002). The anxiety of learning. *Harvard Business Review* 80(3), 100–106.

George, B. (2004). The journey to authenticity. *Leader to Leader* 31, 29–35.

Leider, R. (2004). Is leading your calling? *Leader to Leader* 31, 36–40.

Nash, L. & Stevenson, H. (2004). Sucess that lasts. *Harvard Business Review* 82(2), 102–109.

Offerman, L. R. (2004). When followers become toxic. *Harvard Business Review* 82(1), 54–60.

Vitello-Cicciu, J. M. (2002). Exploring emotional intelligence: Implications for nurse leaders. *JONA* 32(4), 203–209.

Banner Estrella Medical Center (BEMC) Technical and Cultural Interview Guidelines

INTRODUCTION

The hiring process is extremely significant in creating and supporting a culture of health care that will transform the health-care experience. To identify the most qualified applicants, multiple encounters by multiple individuals are believed essential in determining the knowledge, values, and cultural fit of the applicant. The following guidelines are recommended to assist leaders and managers in the selection of BEMC employees.

Basic Interview Steps

1. Human Resource Staff:
   a. Screens candidates for basic qualifications.
   b. Notifies hiring manager of qualified candidates.
   c. Coordinates interview schedule with candidates—Recommended scheduling:

NOTE: Human Resources individual interview scheduled same day as manager interview (45 minutes). The individual interview with hiring manager (30 minutes–1 hour) is scheduled for the same day as Human Resources interview to prevent applicant having to come in twice.

NOTE: Final two applicants will complete steps d & e.

   d. Panel interview of the applicant with 2–3 hiring manager's peers (1 hour)
   e. 3–6 BEMC employees attend an "audition" by the applicant; 15-minute presentation by applicant and 15 minutes for debriefing
2. Hiring manager coordinates with other interviewers on team to determine which behavioral and skills-based questions each person will ask. Balance skills-based and behavioral-based questions during each interview.
3. Hiring manager will prepare applicant for step 3d. by providing an overview of BEMC's culture and vision of "Transforming Health Care for the Future" (fact sheet available to e-mail or give to candidates to help them prepare).

4. During interviews, each interviewer notes the highlights of candidate's responses to questions and completes a "score sheet."
5. After interviews, hiring manager schedules discussion with the interview team to review candidates and make hiring recommendations.

NOTE: Try to keep the same interview team for all candidates interviewed for a single position for consistency.

Banner Estrella Medical Center Selection Tool

There are nine competency categories that will be assessed for the BEMC applicant. Each section includes required questions (in **Bold**) and optional questions. Items can be considered for leaders, clinicians, and staff positions on the basis of the recommendations of the interview design team and are noted in the three columns.

Behavioral Based Competency #1	Leadership
Indicator:	• Provides an environment for people to experience caring, healing, and learning. Treats people with dignity, respect, honesty, and fairness. Recognizes the value of individual differences and the collaboration of people with different strengths and expertise. • Engages people in integrating the Values, Code of Conduct, and Service Standards in daily activities by modeling expected behaviors and reinforcing behaviors demonstrated by others. • Is diligent in efforts to recognize and reward contributions. Provides timely feedback in a constructive manner. Partners with employees to develop meaningful action plans for development.

Questions	Leader	Clinician	Staff
1. Interviewer: Describe the "Environment of Care" for BEMC. Ask: How/why are the values, skills of employees, relationships, and financial accountability included in the leadership role? What experience have you had that connects to this environment?	Yes	No	No
2. What are the core values of your current or former organization? What did you do to ensure your team integrated them into their daily activities? What methods did you use to reinforce desired behaviors? Give me some examples of deliberate attempts on your part to model the values.	Yes	Yes	Yes
3. Delegation is a challenge to many leaders. Describe your process for delegating. How do you know when delegation is not working? How would you improve it and why? Give an example.	Yes	Yes	No
4. Share a time when you provided an employee a unique opportunity to use his/her strengths. What were the circumstances? How did you know this employee could perform the job? How did the system or department improve because of this effort?	Yes	No	No
5. Tell me at least one non-traditional way you provide learning and development to your team. How did this impact your team?	Yes	No	No
6. Describe your most challenging performance assessment. What were the challenges? How did you overcome them? What do you do differently today because of this experience?	Yes	No	No
7. Describe your system for recognizing and rewarding the people on your team. What have you found people most want as rewards and recognition? How did you develop your recognition system?	Yes	No	No

Behavioral Based Competency #2	Achieve Results		
Indicator:	• Business Awareness/Focus: Focuses on quality, cost effectiveness, and services to improve processes and outcomes. Results include streamlined systems and increased patient, customer, and employee satisfaction. • Manages resources: Manages resources efficiently to achieve the best outcomes including people, finances, equipment, materials, and supplies. • Makes values-based and evidence-based business decisions. • Demonstrates commitment to quality and safety.		
		Leader	**Clinician**	**Staff**

Questions	Leader	Clinician	Staff
1. What indicators have been necessary to measure results in your area? Describe your utilization of those indicators in your department's/team's daily operations.	Yes	Yes	No
2. What responsibility have you had with managing the costs of a department or organization? What were the resources in that experience? What did you do to ensure they were used efficiently? How did you know whether or not you were successful?	Yes	No	No
3. Describe a time when you needed to cut costs and you knew your staffing ratio was already very lean. What did you do to realize savings without cutting needed staff? How did the decision impact the business? How did your supervisor respond to your decision?	Yes	No	No
4. What are the areas that you believe are the most important to assuring a safe environment for employees? Patients? Colleagues? Describe a situation in which you improved the safety for one of these groups.	Yes	Yes	Yes
5. Tell me about a process improvement effort you initiated that resulted in improved patient outcomes that was cost effective. What stimulated your effort? What were the steps you took? What were the results or changes in practice/performance that occurred? How did you measure the results? What was the impact on employee satisfaction?	Yes	Yes	Yes
6. How do you evaluate turnover? Is all turnover negative? Why/why not?	Yes	No	No

Behavioral Based Competency #3	Effective Communicator			
Indicator:	• Active listener • Clear, concise verbal and written communication • Effectively manages conflict • Accessible • Follows through			
		Leader	Clinician	Staff
Questions 1. Describe the most significant written document, report, or presentation you have had to complete. How did you pull the information together? What was the response from your target audience?		Yes	Yes	No
2. Having difficult conversations is an essential skill for open and positive environments. How have you learned to: • **Express your own strong feelings** • **Deal with abusive people** • **Deliver difficult decisions to an individual or group** • **Deal with conflict** • **Say no to someone you like**		Yes	Yes	Yes
• **Please give a specific example from your past experience**		Yes	Yes	Yes
3. Describe a time when you realized you needed to make an improvement in your communication skills. How did you manage it?		Yes	Yes	Yes
4. As BEMC is dedicated to advanced computer technology, electronic charting, and wireless communication, employees will need to be competent to work in this environment. Describe your computer/technology skills and how quickly you believe you will adapt to this environment. Also, describe the training that you believe you will need to become competent within one month.		Yes	Yes	Yes
5. In a recent work experience, how have you differentiated appropriate information from inappropriate information to share with patients and customers? Describe the situation. What was the outcome?		Yes	Yes	Yes

Behavioral Based Competency #4	Customer Service
Indicator:	Service Excellence Skills: 1. Treats people he/she serves as guests. Is courteous, makes eye contact, smiles, introduces self, addresses people by name when possible. 2. Presents a professional image. Name badge highly visible. 3. Answers telephone with a smile. Identifies self and asks how he/she can help. 4. Listens to the people we serve and co-workers. Responds promptly and reliably. 5. Anticipates the wants and needs of the people we serve. Asks, "How can I help?" 6. Practices open and honest communication with those with whom he/she serves and works. 7. Keeps the people we serve informed. 8. Maintains a clean and safe environment. 9. Acts to reverse negative service situations using the Anticipate, Acknowledge, Apologize, and Amend service recovery process. 10. Respects the privacy and confidentiality of the people we serve. 11. Strive to master skills needed to do the best for the people we serve. 12. Positively represents BH and BEMC in the workplace and the community.

Questions	Leader	Clinician	Staff
1. **Describe an environment that promotes caring, healing, and learning. Give me an example of an action you've taken to create this type of environment in the workplace.**	Yes	Yes	Yes
2. **Give me an example of a time you provided outstanding customer service.**	Yes	Yes	Yes
3. **Describe a time when you found it difficult to treat a patient or customer as a guest. What was the situation? What made it difficult for you? What did you end up doing?**	Yes	Yes	Yes
4. Think of a recent situation in which you were able to identify customer's or patient's needs before he/she asked for help. What did you do? What was the patient's response?	Yes	Yes	Yes
5. How have you handled negative customer situations? How have you calmed an angry or upset patient/visitor/coworker? Cite a specific example.	Yes	Yes	Yes
6. What would make you proud of the way we treat our patients?	Yes	Yes	Yes

Behavioral Based Competency #5	Teamwork		
Indicator:	• Understands and incorporates "relational wholeness" into actions (avoids silo behavior) • Collaborative: Takes opportunities to work with others to find solutions to problems • Accountable: Follows through on commitments • Becomes a resource for other team members • Plays to own strengths and stretches out of comfort zone in team interactions • Shares information so others may be successful • Supports groups' solutions to problems		
	Leader	**Clinician**	**Staff**
Questions 1. **Tell me about the last time you collaborated on a project with others. What were the circumstances? Who was involved? What did you do to contribute?**	Yes	Yes	Yes
2. **Under what circumstances is it difficult to be cooperative on a team? Describe a time when you've faced these challenges. How did you handle them? How did it turn out?**	Yes	Yes	Yes
3. Tell me about a team decision in your current or past position that you were not in agreement with. What was the decision? What was your idea that wasn't used? How did you respond to the decision? What did you do to demonstrate support of the decision even though you did not agree with it?	Yes	Yes	Yes
4. How would members of your most recent team describe you?	Yes	Yes	Yes
5. What prevents people from sharing information or skills with others? What have you done to overcome these barriers?	Yes	Yes	Yes
6. Coaching is about providing feedback for growth, improvement, and/or correction. Describe your skills with each situation. Tell me about a time you've used these skills well.	Yes	Yes	Yes

Behavioral Based Competency #6	Personal Attributes: Job Fit		
Indicator:	• Energized • Confidence • Respectful • Open • Fun-loving • Creative • Honest		
	Leader	**Clinician**	**Staff**
Questions 1. Describe how you have gone about developing an environment that promotes caring, healing, and learning. Please be specific. What were the circumstances? What did you do? What were the results?	Yes	Yes	Yes
2. How can you help BEMC transform the health-care experience? Give specific examples.	Yes	Yes	Yes
3. How do you treat others with dignity, respect, honesty, and fairness? Please provide a specific example.	Yes	Yes	Yes
4. Have you ever had the opportunity to work in an "Open Architecture," cubicle-type environment? If yes, give me an example of how you worked in that environment. What worked well? What didn't work so well? If no, what types of issues might you have working in this type of environment and how would you handle these issues?	Yes	Yes	Yes
5. Tell me about your greatest professional accomplishment. What made it especially challenging? What type of feedback did you receive? What makes you the most proud of this?	Yes	Yes	Yes
6. If you took out an ad in the *New York Times* and had to describe yourself in only three words, what would those words be and why?	Yes	Yes	Yes
7. Describe your ideal work environment.	Yes	Yes	Yes
8. Tell me about a work situation that irritated you. What did you do?	Yes	Yes	Yes
9. What responsibilities do you want and what kinds of results do you expect to achieve in your next job?	Yes	Yes	Yes

Behavioral Based Competency #7	Problem Solving & Creativity			
Indicator:	• Seeks variety of alternatives/approaches • Identifies variety of sources • Solves problems effectively • Can articulate a problem solving process • Takes calculated risks • Critical thinking skills—confidence, flexibility, intuition, open-mindedness, perseverance, questioning, and reflection			
		Leader	Clinician	Staff
Questions 1. How do you define critical thinking? Give me an example of a non-routine or more difficult problem you had to solve. How did you work through to a solution?		Yes	Yes	Yes
2. Tell me about a time when you did your best, but were unable to solve a problem. What were the barriers? What did you do to remove them? What did you learn from the experience?		Yes	Yes	Yes
3. Give an example of a situation in which you took a calculated risk in a recent position. What were your considerations? What was the outcome?		Yes	Yes	Yes
4. Please describe the last creative solution you came up with in response to a problem. What was the problem? How did you work through to your solution?		Yes	Yes	Yes

Behavioral Based Competency #8	Manages Change		
Indicator:	• Manages ambiguity • Understands behaviors and change management techniques and theory • Asks questions so he/she can support decisions. Does not resist changes in the organization. • Communicates throughout change process		
	Leader	**Clinician**	**Staff**
Questions 1. **Tell me about a recent change in your workplace. What did you do to learn more about the rationale for the change? What did you learn? How did it affect your ability to manage the change?**	Yes	Yes	Yes
2. When was the last time you initiated a major change in your life? Please provide a specific example. What drove your decision to make the change? What did you do to ensure the change went as you expected it to?	Yes	Yes	Yes
3. Describe a work situation in which a project you worked on and felt was important was delayed or postponed due to other changes in the organization. How did you handle this situation?	Yes	Yes	Yes

Behavioral Based Competency #9	Manages Time/Sets Priorities		
Indicator:	• Organized • Manages multiple projects effectively • Meets deadlines with quality work		
	Leader	**Clinician**	**Staff**
Questions 1. Tell me about your work experience in managing multiple job priorities with varied deadlines. When and how do you determine priority and deadline changes?	Yes	Yes	Yes
2. You are on the phone with another department resolving a problem. The intercom pages you for a customer on hold. Your manager returns your monthly report with red pen markings and demands corrections within the hour. What do you do?	Yes	Yes	Yes
3. Think of a typical day when you had plenty of things to do. Describe how you scheduled your time.	Yes	Yes	Yes

BEMC Interview Guide
Summary Sheet for Leadership Roles

Date of Interview:

Candidate Name:

Position:

Interviewer:

Competency Categories	(1–5 Score) 1 = unacceptable 2 = below average 3 = meets minimal expectations 4 = above average 5 = outstanding	Question Number(s)	Candidate Responses
Leadership			
Achieves Results			
Effective Communicator			
Customer Service			
Teamwork			
Personal Attributes: Job Fit			
Creativity & Risk Taking			
Manages Change			
Manages Time/Sets Priorities			
TOTAL SCORE			

Would you recommend this person for hire?

If yes, what are the key reasons for hiring this person?

If no, what are the key reasons for not hiring?

Contact Kathy.Stanley@Bannerhealth.com or Connie.Harmsen@Bannerhealth.com
for additional information on the interview guide.

Turning Toxic Behaviors into Transformational Actions

CHAPTER OBJECTIVES:

Upon completion of this chapter, the reader will:

1. Differentiate between healthy and toxic leader behaviors.

2. Examine selected behaviors of new employee hazing, destructive confidants, poor communication and feedback dysfunction as sources of toxicity in the organization.

3. Formulate at least three strategies to decrease toxic behaviors as a developing Quantum leader.

4. Critique the value of story telling as a meaningful leader strategy.

INTRODUCTION: HEALING IS OUR BUSINESS

Healing is our business, and yet not all health-care leadership practices result in outcomes that reflect therapeutic intentions. Many outcomes are in fact quite negative and detrimental to not only individuals and teams but also the organization as a whole. In this chapter, sources of toxicity that are specific to the health-care marketplace, organizational structure, individual behaviors, and team processes will be examined, along with strategies for eliminating toxic practices and replacing them with therapeutic behaviors more reflective of the healer.

TOXICITY IS . . .

Healthy behaviors seldom get the attention that toxic behaviors or negative outcomes receive. Consider the question often posed by nurses, "What is most evident when it is missing?" The response is *nursing*. When nursing is being practiced in healthy and meaningful ways, the attention it receives is minimal compared to when nursing does not occur as expected. When there is shortage of nurses, nursing care cannot be delivered in the same way as when there were more nurses. Shortages lead to lack of care, missed treatments, low morale, high turnover, and ultimately high costs to consumers. Understanding the optimal way health

---

Gem
A toxin is a substance or poison that has an inherent tendency to impair health and destroy life.

Impact of Nursing Shortages

• Patient mortality	Aiken, 1994; Cho, 2003
• Length of stay	ANA 1997; Flood & Diers, 1998; Pronovost, 1999
• Medication errors	ANA Report Card; Blegen & Vaughn, 1998; Patient Safety, USP Reviews
• Nosocomial pneumonia	ANA 1997; Blegen et al, 1998
• Turnover	VHA, 2002
• Failure to rescue	Aiken, 2003
• Cost to consumer	McCue, 2003

care should be provided, as well as what happens when the outcomes are less than optimal, can help us determine when healthy processes become toxic and negatively impact health-care service.

SOURCES OF TOXICITY

Toxicity in organizations seldom occurs obviously or in resoundingly strong practices and behaviors. Organizational toxicity is often subtle and seemingly insignificant as it spreads its highly venomous substance, destroying the essence of health and healing cultures. Toxicity seldom results from one source or a single activity; it is a consequence of several factors and pressures that once understood can be reversed by the collective actions of competent leaders.

The Marketplace

Failure to provide service of the highest quality in the eyes of the consumer, regardless of social or economic status, personal attributes, or the nature of health problems has been identified as the most significant ethical issue encountered in health-care organizations (Cooper, 2002). Marketplace forces seriously challenge the ability of the leader to achieve and sustain financial viability. The chosen strategies to achieve organizational goals may compromise the essential work of the organization, namely, providing effective, value-based health-care services. Thus, from seemingly good intentions, negative, toxic outcomes result. The organization may be financially solvent, yet patient care outcomes are marginal and health-care workers are disenfranchised, angry, and often leave the organization searching for less toxic and healthier organizations.

Organizational Structure

The pathways for communication and decision making in organizations can be a subtle but significant source of toxicity. When the organization espouses shared leadership and yet reinforces practices of double-checking others believed entrusted with the power and authority to make decisions, the situation is in conflict. The message of this double standard diminish the integrity of organizational leadership and trust among employees and creates more toxicity. What a conundrum when professional nurses believe they are members of a shared leadership council with decision-making accountability and authority and yet the decisions they make are changed or overridden without their input. In many organizations, shared leadership councils are created below the traditional executive leadership team chaired by the chief executive officer. The executive team reviews all council decisions and often overrides or redirects councils to shift or reconsider decisions. This approach creates confusion for council participants and discourages future participation. In time, employees are demoralized, and trusting relationships are forever undermined.

TOXIC INDIVIDUAL BEHAVIORS

Not all toxicity can be attributed to the organizational structure. While poorly designed and ineffective systems make it difficult for good individuals to do good things, the need exists for leaders to take action to assure that both the individual and the system are examined for potential shortcomings. System policies and procedures, computer system effectiveness, reward strategies, and individual behaviors require analysis prior

---

Quantum Discussion

"Healing NOT" Behaviors

In your workgroup, identify those behaviors that are believed to be healing, but in reality are NOT. How can you begin to eliminate such behaviors and replace them with more appropriate behaviors for a health-care organization?

Examples include:
- Withholding feedback/key information
- Smiling sarcasm
- The "Devil's Advocate" role

to choosing a correcting strategy. Denial and resistance to examining current system attributes will serve only as ineffective rationalization and will avoid addressing the fundamental issue.

Individuals within organizations may fail to embrace established values and cultural norms for several reasons. These reasons or rationalizations are related to system functioning, but the accountability for behavior rests squarely with the individual. Hofman (2004) identified seven reasons why good people behave badly.

1. *Lack of organizational loyalty.* Often short-term employees have not established allegiance to the organization but merely are earning a paycheck. High staff turnover further contributes to such behaviors and lack of commitment to the organization.
2. *Pressure to succeed as defined by the organization.* Some organizations have placed emphasis on net income above clinical outcomes and value conformity over candor, resulting in personnel who act inappropriately and unethically. The recent fraud and abuse violations of several national health-care systems was most likely motivated by an overemphasis on financial criteria.
3. *Rules are for the others.* Driving five miles above the speed limit to get to an important meeting on time, believing that one's business is more important than following rules, is a simple example of this behavior. Certain employees assert that they should not be subject to certain policies and procedures.
4. *Believing their actions are not illegal.* Being ethical is more than being compliant with statutory regulations. Not every action or behavior is governed by statute, nor should they be. Yet, some believe that ethical acts and legal acts are synonymous. To be sure, there are many unethical actions that are not legislated.
5. *Pressure from peers.* The combination of strong-willed colleagues with those who are inexperienced, easily influenced by others, or conflict avoiders sets up conditions for toxic behaviors. Acquiescing to overbearing colleagues diminishes the probability for effective dialogue and high quality decision making.
6. *Lack of resources.* Much like the pressure-to-succeed behavior, when resources are limited individuals attempt to cut corners as an excuse for unsatisfactory work rather than work to adjust demands to more closely match available resources. Eliminating safety evaluations and safety measures are examples of cutting corners inappropriately.
7. *A sense of entitlement.* An inflated sense of self-importance and an absence of organizational pride contribute to the belief that the organization or the community owes one something. An example of entitlement abuse can be the use of earned sick time. In those organizations that have separate sick hours benefits, employees often use the sick time at will rather than solely for sickness in order to not lose the earned time.

New Employee Hazing: Tolerating Change Avoidance

When leaders do not walk their talk, do not live the values and policies they endorse, yet still speak to these values from the podium, members of the organization recognize the inconsistency and interpret the actions as a serious lack of integrity. Frequently, leaders assume new positions with expectations to take the department to a higher and more productive level. Everyone in the interviewing process agrees that changes are needed and needed quickly. However, something very different occurs.

Discussion

Ineffective System Processes

Consider the following routine interactions in most health-care settings. Each process has at some point in your career been identified as less than optimal.

- patient admission
- acquiring capital equipment

Discuss each process from the perspective of supporting policies and procedures, computer system support adequacy, and individual competencies to perform the processes.

- What is working?
- What changes would make the process more timely and value-based?

Discussion

Rules for Others

List the rules or policies that are routinely ignored without consequences.

What actions should be taken to decrease the noncompliance?

- Reinforce the value of the policy and expectations?
- Modify the policy?
- Eliminate the policy?

Examples to consider for discussion:

- Hand washing
- Returning from breaks on time
- Documentation
- Eating in designated areas

Discussion

New Employee Hazing Assessment

Meet with the last five individuals hired in your organization. Discuss their expectations and what really happened. If the expectations are not close to reality, discuss what happened and how to reduce the gap.

Eliminate employee hazing!

As new employees join organizations, a subtle but toxic process may occur: *employee hazing.* This situation of toxic mentoring follows the selection and hiring of the new employees. Although leaders overtly believe that innovative ideas are the lifeblood of any organization, especially in today's rapidly changing health-care environment, obstacles are often covertly placed in the way of new employee innovation. After intense rounds of interviews, the candidate with the best believed fit with the vision of the organization is hired and touted as the key to future success.

The new leader joins the organization and is quickly met with messages and guidance that are intended to assist in the orientation and socialization process but provide obstacles to those innovative ideas on the very first day of employment! New leaders are told of the failures of the past, why certain strategies did not work, or current policies and regulations that would make it impossible to consider innovative ideas. Current employees reflect on long-held traditions, the need to ensure peaceful relationships, the importance of not upsetting long-term employees who have given so much to the company, and finally the need to go slowly in introducing and implementing any changes to assure employee support and buy-in. Seldom are new leaders met with passionate optimism and enthusiasm to figure out how to test new ideas in the face of the established organizational culture.

When the organization is not getting individuals with the new and truly innovative ideas necessary to stay ahead of the competition, the organizational culture and norms may be hazing the innovation out of them. Examination of organizational policies and procedures specific to orientation of new employees is essential. Inclusion of expectations to bring innovative ideas rather than expectations of blind acceptance with cultural norms is the first step to the elimination of hazing and support for innovation.

Destructive Confidants

Organizational toxicity may also emanate from destructive confidants. Traditional leaders avoid any hint of dependency on others, yet the need for a close confidant is rooted in childhood, the need to feel close to someone, to feel understood, cared for, and loved. Having a trusted confidant with whom to discuss challenging issues, share fears and experiences, and gain unfiltered advice adds to the leader's competence. Given the isolated position of the leader, selecting a confidant deserves special attention to ensure that the goals and motives of the confidant are congruent. Too often, individuals in the organization shelter the leader from unpleasant or conflicting information. Executive coaching programs can be designed to assist leaders is recognizing the values and pitfalls of confidants.

According to Sulkowicz (2004), many confidants end up hurting, undermining, or otherwise exploiting CEOs when they are at their most vulnerable. Although intentions may be honorable on the surface, confidants become close friends who affirm the leader, rather than serving to challenge and sharpen the leader's effectiveness and keeping the leader's best interest at the forefront. When a confidant becomes dangerous, the leader is often the last one to know when and how the relationship became toxic. Admitting that the relationship is toxic further demoralizes the already isolated and vulnerable leader.

Consider the situation in which a confidant preys on the leader's anxieties about certain competitors, relationships with others in the community, and personal characteristics. Rather than challenge the reality of the anxiety, the toxic confidant reinforces the hopelessness of the nega-

---

Quantum Tip

Eliminating New Employee Hazing

- Avoid the tendency to "correct" new employees into the current culture.
- Encourage new ideas. At the end of each day, ask new employees what observations they have made and potential changes that could benefit the organization.
- Evaluate your own behaviors:
  - How long does it take new employees to look and act like everyone else?
  - In what subtle ways have you "doused" new employee ideas?

Quantum Point

Three Destructive Confidants

Reflectors—Confidants who mirror the leader

Insulators—Prevent critical information from getting out or getting in

Usurpers—Confidant who ingratiates him- or herself with leader in a desperate bid for power

Sulkowicz, 2004

tive relationship or the potential for further negative actions. Another situation is in the selection of key members of the leadership team. Destructive confidants reinforce selection of less competent members to assure they are not exposed. Selecting those with less experience, less education, and less competence under the guise of mentoring severely limits the organization's capacity for innovation and growth.

Avoiding these destructive relationships may seem impossible for many leaders, given the often narcissistic role of the leader. Yet these narcissistic behaviors are also essential in creating, achieving, and sustaining organizational visions. To minimize the destructive confidant syndrome, several strategies are worth examining. Watch for the warning signs of a destructive relationship:

- Employees complain that you are not accessible
- You feel no one but your confidant understands you
- Your confidant discourages you from getting other opinions or counsel

These signs may be reflective of a larger problem as well, such as procrastination, mediocre communication skills, or lack of trust in others by the leader.

Effective leaders develop many confidants or colleagues whom they trust, and value their wisdom rather than a single confidant. Having only one confidant can be stunting and immobilizing for the leader who desires realistic mentoring for dialogue and reflection. When leaders hear only positive feedback, the alarm should sound and the search for confidants to represent complex dimensions of health-care leadership should begin in earnest.

Communication Gone Awry

Communication among employees, patients, and physicians has long been a challenge for organizations. Delivering the right message to the right person, at the right time, with the right intent does not occur consistently for a variety of reasons. The rationale for delivering partial or poorly timed messages is often due to impulsive or spontaneous actions that simply override good sense! The challenge to continue to work toward effective communication remains with all individuals.

Abuse of Power: Verbal Abuse

Abusive communication is not always expressed loudly and profanely. Often, verbal abuse is in the form of a believed "kind and generous" sharing of information. Much attention has been given to overt disruptive behavior in organizations.

Abuse of Power: Decision Making

Leaders often abuse power in their eagerness to remedy system imperfections. Efforts become aggressive and nonparticipatory when the issue is believed to be critical and urgent.

Toxic Mentoring

The need to create succession plans for future leadership often serves as a vehicle for toxicity, continuing those practices that are no longer effective and even detrimental to organizational creativity and energy. While not overtly toxic, mentors may emphasize the continuation of

---

Discussion

Uncommon Verbal Abuse

This statement was made by a smiling supervisor in the presence of patients and co-workers: "It's hard to believe that with your experience and skills, you did not provide the information to this family. I'm sure that you will take care of this quickly." It is disrespectful, confrontational, and demeaning without the typical "aura" of verbal abuse.

Identify 3 situations in which verbal abuse occurred that did not involve yelling, arrogance, profanity or physical threats.

What strategies can you identify to address these behaviors and to avoid them in the future?

Decision-Making Characteristics

Traditional

- Compartmentalism
- Focus on analysis to determine cause and effect
- Standardization of processes
- Emphasis on structure and process
- Individual leaders dominate
- Control mechanisms to minimize variation

Shared Leadership

- Collaboration
- Synthesis of ideas
- Teamwork
- Collective wisdom: Recognition of individual strengths as contributions to the whole
- Attention to the whole system
- Emphasis on value-based outcomes

previous practices that were controlling and reinforced the hierarchical nature of a command and control decision-making model. These behaviors unintentionally serve to reinforce past practices that were appropriate for the industrial age. Believing that such strategies are also effective for the information age belies the reality of the new age and all of its characteristics. The past is reinforced as appropriate, and the future is denied.

Consider the situation in which a leader believes that five years of experience is required to understand and function in a particular position. A candidate for the position has two years of experience, and the desire to serve in the role, the confidence, and the technical and relational competence, but not the five years of experience. Current leaders encourage the candidate to gain the experience and then apply for the position. The traditional time for "paying one's dues" is sustained, and the opportunity to coach and mentor a strong candidate is missed. Mentors from outside the organization may be more appropriate than current leaders from within. When a mentor can be objective about situations without the historical bias of the organization, the leader learns to challenge existing practices and structures in the journey of leadership. To be sure, new leaders do not need to change everything but rather need to clearly know the rationale for existing practices and become comfortable learning when to sustain practices that are effective.

Managing the Unmanageable Leader

Not all leaders are competent in their positions. Employees who are not getting along with their leader are often challenged to get along or move on. Before moving on in utter frustration or just tolerating the incompetence, they should give serious consideration to other options. Even when your leader is the clone of every disastrous leader you have ever read about, heard about, or had nightmares about, or before things really get out of hand, the following steps are recommended to assist employees in making wise decisions.

1. Meet with him or her and clarify what is expected in terms of style of getting the job done. The priorities of your former boss and current boss may be very different in basic work methods.
2. Carefully confront criticism in private. Express your desire to communicate effectively, discuss your negative perceptions of the interaction, and finally ask for guidance in how to communicate effectively with him or her (no matter how difficult it is!).
3. Check the mirror! Your own attitude may be part of the problem. Have you been helpful since this new person joined your organization? Stand-offish? Annoyed? Neutral, neither negative nor helpful? Is your body language outrageously loud? Are facial expressions and tone of your voice telling of your dissatisfaction?
4. Reflect on the issues. Is your shadow showing? The style, mannerisms, and communications that annoy us the most are often behaviors of our own that we ourselves struggle to manage.
5. Make your decision. Do not dawdle as the toxicity may only increase.

Feedback Dysfunction

Gaining an understanding of what others are thinking is essential to good communication and teamwork. Often coworkers become caught up in the need to share their feelings openly and honestly, and the result is less than satisfactory. Communications are interpreted as whining or complaining without purpose or accountability. Perceptions of personal attacks, global commentaries on vague issues, opinionating about conditions not under one's control, and failing to address issues to the appropriate person result in toxic communication. These communications serve no useful purpose, waste valuable organizational time, and too often are no more than idle gossip destructive to the culture.

TOXIC TEAM PROCESSES

In the best of all worlds, the processes that emerge in organizations are the result of deliberately designed authority and decision-making structures and are then embraced and practiced by the individuals in the organization. Given the realities of organizational dynamics, which includes the recency of the structure design, the match of individual skill sets to the established vision and values, and the personal motivation of each leader to actively support the defined culture, disconnects between what is stated and what is practiced occur, all too often resulting in toxic conditions.

Consider the organization that has designed shared leadership structures but does not always achieve the processes to support these structures. Shared leadership council structures have been identified and created. The need for member skills of collaboration, negotiation, and facilitation, and the ability to surrender the once-required strong, authoritarian ego are also agreed to and included in performance expectations. In reality, decision making is offered to councils but is often overridden, negated, or ignored. Recommendations by councils are seldom integrated into organizational policy, thus rendering the work of councils insignificant.

SOURCES OF TOXICITY: TEAM PROCESSES

Shared Decision Making: Rhetoric or Reality

Toxic behaviors can be present in decision-making processes. Transitional leaders or those leaders who began their careers in organizations steeped in command and control require significant support in moving to a shared leadership model. Ongoing dialogue and reflection are essential to ensure that all members of the team are in fact living in the new participative model. McMurry (2003) notes that often leaders become overenchanted with participative processes, yet still operate from an autocratic model.

McMurry (2003) describes three types of leadership: group autocracy, blind autocracy, and benevolent autocracy. They can be very subtle but highly toxic to the organization. The phenomenon of group autocracy typically occurs in large, bureaucratic organizations in which strategic decisions are not *officially* made by the leader, who lacks courage and takes refuge in the principle of unanimity. The leader maintains bureaucratic autocracy without leadership, imagination, or drive while functioning under the guise of shared leadership.

As health-care leaders transition from autocratic behaviors to leading from a shared perspective, with the expectations to produce optimal results, respond quickly, and assure positive employee satisfaction, there is a tendency to subtly slip into group autocracy behaviors. In essence, leaders are preaching shared decision making yet operating as autocrats.

Both blind autocracy and benevolent autocracy behaviors belie the guiding principles and values of shared leadership. Leaders firmly

---

Quantum Tip

Effective Feedback: Personal Expectations

1. Create expectations for regular feedback sessions.
2. Be proactive: Avoid procrastination in addressing issues.
3. Avoid the tendency to deny issues.
4. Avoid brooding.
5. Respond to positive feedback appreciatively; do not minimize accomplishments.
6. Respond to negative feedback slowly; request clarification and validation of issues.
7. Request recommendations for different approaches.
8. Determine if changes are appropriate for you.
9. Implement new behaviors or renegotiate issues.

Tips for Effective Feedback: Managing Others

1. Establish formal and informal review processes. Monthly discussions should be the minimum frequency for feedback.
2. Address potential fear of feedback issues. Create expectations for open and honest communication.
3. Avoid the tendency of providing superficial feedback. Provide objective feedback specific to established goals.
4. Avoid angry confrontations, defensiveness, ambivalent conversations.

---

3 Types of Decision-Making Autocracy

Group Autocracy: Decisions discussed by the group, but in reality made by the leader who is "hiding" in the group process.

Blind Autocracy: Decisions made by the leader who directs others to trust his or her decisions due to the competence of the leader.

Benevolent Autocracy: Decisions made by the leader on the assumption that others cannot make optimal and effective decisions in a team setting.

R. McMurray

Toxic vs. Humanistic Values

Toxic	**Humanistic**
• Overcontrol	• Trusting
• Reminding of past failures	• Focus on new approaches to improve the past
• Identifying mistakes	• Valuing unsuccessful attempts
• Double-checking work	• Expecting personal accountability
• Controlling processes	

Decision Making

Unilateral

• Following laws
• Facility licensure requirements
• Nurse Practice Act
• Accreditation requirements

Shared

• Processes to meet laws, licensure requirements, Nurse Practice Act, and accreditation requirements

entrenched in autocratic practices believe that, although the democratic participative philosophy of management is more productive in the long term, stimulates creativity and development, and improves morale, the probability of such behaviors succeeding is minimal. Lower and middle managers have not been given opportunities to demonstrate shared leadership practices, making the prospects for this new model of leadership negligible. Current managers are dependent upon strong autocratic leaders to provide specific direction and appear insecure and ineffective. Thus, leaders assume that the only way to get the work done is to create a benevolent autocracy model of leadership. The lack of emerging behaviors from lower and middle managers requires the autocrat to continue with the current behaviors.

To shift from this dehumanizing and toxic model, leaders are required to transition to a new and more humanistic approach that values the contributions of each employee as the more appropriate vehicle to higher organizational performance. Not surprising, this transition requires time, energy, and patience, which are not always readily given to the process.

Black, White, or Neither or Both?

Another source of toxicity can be found when the zeal to implement shared leadership overrides common sense. The notion that the only way to work is through teams can be problematic. Embedded in a shared leadership model are the expectations that at certain times group participation in decision making is not possible and members of the team must make autocratic decisions in certain situations. Attempting to live in the absoluteness of one style or the other creates uncertainty and toxicity in the organization. When employees are expecting one process exclusively and then experience several processes, the trust level within the organizations declines dramatically. It is the allegiance to the defined values and mission of the organization that must remain the constant in all decisions, regardless of the decision-making process.

Toxicity emerges when the council structures are mere window dressing and decisions continue to be made autocratically on the basis of inconsistently defined values, not only at the executive level but also at the unit level. Most importantly, toxicity can be reversed by clarifying council charter expectations for work to be managed and outcomes to be achieved.

A recent situation resulting from the failure to distinguish unilateral from shared decision making involved an emergency department. The state department was conducting a survey, following a complaint from a patient who believed she suffered unnecessary pain in the emergency room. Upon investigation, the complaint was not substantiated. However, the state department was duty-bound to cite the organization for failing to follow its own policy on pain management. The unilateral decision from the state required each department to have a policy specific to pain management for patients in the emergency department. The department director created a policy and an expectation for nurses to assess ten factors related to pain for each patient upon admission and upon discharge. During the review of records, zero compliance with the facility policy was noted; thus, the facility was cited. While some may believe that regulatory agencies impose unreasonable and bureaucratic standards, it is often the organization that has "overinterpreted" the standard. The unilateral state requirement is non-negotiable. The processes and content developed by the organization to meet this requirement should be developed by the team to reflect the nature of the patient care in each department.

Covert Greed or Competition Gone Bad

Within leadership teams, the enthusiasm for success can often move beyond reasonable success to that for greed. Greed is a trait that we typically attribute to others, as it is a profoundly negative quality. Given that money and things are often considered measures of success, the desperation to acquire things can become toxic not only in one's personal life but also in the workplace. When individuals become aggressive and manipulative in acquiring goods and money, the behaviors become pathological greed (Contu, 2003).

Recent events in corporate America have exposed the negative outcomes of greed. Chief executive officers have desperately worked to amass more and more fortune for unknown reasons. Fortunately, greed is tempered by social norms and can be harnessed to serve social ends. In less than 50 years, the management of hospitals and health systems has shifted from a passive, custodial, and largely benign administrative tradition to an aggressive, growth-oriented, entrepreneurial management framework (Goldsmith, 1998). Not surprising, the economic position of health-care systems has also improved significantly with the new technologies and the transition from primarily inpatient services to multisite ambulatory settings.

The desire for the success can become toxic or be considered unhealthy greed when the desire for more profits and more buildings overshadows the fundamental need for preservation of the health-care mission and organizational survival. Traditionally, the profoundly negative essence of greed has not been associated with health-care services. Yet, increasing numbers of organizations prioritize shareholder gain as the priority. When expectations and reward structures designed to support primarily shareholder gain drive decision making, the chasm between leaders and professionals is enlarged; as leaders discard the core accountabilities of quality health-care services in favor of personal gain, greed of a very unholy nature exists! In some cases, not-for-profit organizations are also at risk for unholy greed. The desire for more equipment, more technology, more physical locations, and higher net income margins can easily create toxic conditions. In the health-care marketplace, there will never be enough dollars to provide the highest quality patient care, the most progressive technology, and the newest physical settings. Yet, some leaders work to achieve these goals at the expense of providing value-based health-care services.

It is no surprise that this success has an undesired outcome; of the alienation of professionals who are the lifeblood of health care and who bear most of the moral risk of the health-care transaction. The cultural disintegration resulting from organizational greed has impacted nurses, physicians, technicians, and social workers, who see themselves transformed into commodities and marginalized by the corporate culture of health care services. The chasm between leaders and professionals remains, while financial strength is at its peak and expansion abounds. The tension of this paradox is certainly recognized by leaders and providers, yet the hostility remains as health-care systems continue to grow to the point of dwarfing both the patient and the caregiver who must work within them. Some organizations have grown beyond human scale and have lost their focus on the daily life-and-death struggles occurring within their walls, thus fueling toxicity.

Greed can be seen not only in health-care leaders but also in patients who believe they are entitled to every medical treatment known to man, even without evidence of probable success of such treatments or commitment to therapeutic supportive behaviors. In many situations, patient advocacy and informed consent that clearly delineates all of the

---

Quantum Point

Tempering Greed Assessment

1. Assess your motives for new projects—is it for personal recognition, contributions to the industry, or solely to make money?
2. Are the mission and values of the organization congruent with the work of the organization?
3. Is the organization achieving the best possible outcomes, or are more resources needed at the bedside to assure excellence?
4. Is consideration given to the Earth's limited resources?
5. Does a spirit of altruism permeate the health-care organization and its work?

True Success Characteristics

- Values are clear and known to others.
- Service to the public is achieved.
- Resources are used appropriately.
- Services are value-based and make a difference in health care outcomes.
- Integrity is never challenged.

advantages and disadvantages can assist patients and their families in making more realistic decisions.

Personal greed and selfishness often transfer to the workplace and interfere with group commitment and willingness to take appropriate action. Individuals gauge decisions on the basis of their personal wants, at the expense of effective team collaboration and decision making. Decisions that ought to be good for patient care are not made, in favor of personal expectations of obtaining more time off and more overtime pay than is reasonable.

Health-care workers can be guilty of greed in the expectations of excessive benefits and hourly wages. Employees may be caught up in the situation or strongly influenced by a labor organization to always ask for more from an employer without a corresponding contribution. Channeling greed to constructive purposes is a necessary leadership skill that is seldom recognized or articulated. Assisting employees to understand the marketplace value that each contributes (or does not contribute) as well as competitive wages and benefits within the industry elevates wage and benefits discussions to a much higher and more appropriate level. Employees must first know what difference they make to the organization's mission before demanding more from the employer. Further, when employees clearly understand their role and importance in the organization, morale is increased and efforts to continually enhance those contributions occur in a much healthier manner.

Valuing Fragmented or Partial Leadership

Organizational toxicity can increase when good and effective leadership is equated with partial leadership skills. Strength in *some* areas of leadership does not make a quantum leader. It is no secret that some expert technicians do not possess expert relationship skills, or that some leaders have outstanding relationship skills and little ability to envision and lead a team through health care's challenges. It is also not a secret that these individuals hold and sustain significant leadership positions and continue to demonstrate only partial leadership competence.

For example, the nurse executive with exceptional financial management skills may not possess exceptional or even average relationship skills. This nurse executive is continually rewarded for financial performance while employee satisfaction ratings are less than average, resulting in high turnover. Valuing of partial leadership by senior leaders can be acceptable for the short term but disastrous in the long term. Partial leadership erodes trust and negates the values of holism, values that form the essential patient care experience and include physical, social, financial, and technical components.

Arizona Nurse Leadership Model

Recognizing the limitations of current health care leadership models, nurse leaders in Arizona developed the Arizona Nurse Leadership (ANL) Model to offer a comprehensive approach, which included six essential competencies of the quantum leader for the information age (Malloch, 2003). This model defines skills of nursing as managing relationships; communicating the role and contribution of nursing; creating effective working environments; impacting public policy; defining the value of nursing in marketplace language; and assuring that the work of nursing is in concert with the mission of health care. These skills form the framework of the larger model that encompasses the traditional activities of coaching, mentoring, and facilitating. The lack of these highly developed

---

Leadership: Examples of Partial vs. Comprehensive

Partial	Comprehensive
• Highly competent in clinical and relationship skills; poor governance skills	• Highly competent in clinical, relational, financial, conceptual, and governance skills
• Excellent manager of technical aspects; poor financial skills	• Able to identify ongoing needs to continually enhance skills
• Excellent financial and productivity management skills; poor conceptual and interpersonal skills	• Able to coach and mentor others to achieve comprehensive leadership skills

---

Arizona Nurse Leadership Competencies

• Conceptual	• Political
• Technical	• Commercial
• Interpersonal	• Governance

skills in leadership roles leads to frustration, disenfranchisement from the health-care organization, partial leadership, and, all too often, resignation from the health-care system. The six competencies of the ANL model, based on the work of Longest (1998) are described in the next section. These characteristics are requirements for not only leaders, but also staff nurses and nurse educators.

Conceptual competence includes both the knowledge and skill to envision one's place in the organization and within the larger society. The leader must be able to visualize the interrelationships that exist in workplaces and to integrate the cultural and historical development of values, beliefs, and norms of nursing within the workplace. Clear articulation of the role of nursing and its fit within the organization provides for the visible yet integrated role of nursing in the provision of health care.

From the staff nurse to the manager to the leader to the educator, the ability to model the vision for nursing is fundamental. Recognizing its historical development, leaders must continually evaluate, modify, and connect the role of nursing to the realities of the social, economic, and political environment. The understanding of the conceptual fit of nursing with society serves to assist the leader in clearly articulating these interactions and accountabilities. Living by the ANA Social Policy Statement and knowing the contributions of nursing to the health of society and the cost of nursing care are some of the essential conceptual competencies of the nurse leader.

Technical competence of leaders encompasses those skills and knowledge specific to planning, designing, evaluating, and measuring performance. Specifically, technical competence encompasses the skills the nurse leader must have to ensure that nursing care is provided in the environment for which she or he is accountable. These skills are the fundamental work of leaders and are often believed to be the majority of the required skills, rather than only one facet of the role. Too often, the emphasis is placed primarily on technical skills at the expense of the integrated leadership skill set.

The technically competent leader is able to use problem-solving skills at the team level, understands the psychology of work satisfaction that translates into commitment, retention, and high productivity, and is able to measure performance based on established goals and standards. Also within the technical competence realm is the ability to create an environment for employees that is safe, challenges them to think critically, and encourages professional development and innovation.

Interpersonal competence embodies the knowledge and skill of human interactions and relations through which one leads other people in pursuit of common objectives. The ability to form collaborative relationships among caregivers, patients, and community members in the provision of care as well as in socializing others to the profession cannot be overstated. Forming relationships is the cornerstone of healing services, and nurses must be experts in this area. Nurses must relate effectively with patients, other health-care professionals, members of the community, and the formal organizations of nursing to assure that the role of the nurse is explicitly enacted in the social setting as defined in the social policy of nursing.

Expertise in interpersonal competence for nurse leaders includes the expectation that the current knowledge of the profession is represented and personal development is self-directed to remain contemporary with the profession. The link with not only individuals and teams but also the profession of nursing embodies relationship expertise for nurse leaders. Nurses with expertise in interpersonal relationship building are respected

---

Conceptual Competence Checklist

1. Am I able to articulate where nursing services fit within my organization? In my community?
2. Does the vision for nursing reflect the defined fit of nursing?
3. Do principles of systems thinking and systems analysis serve to further explain the complex dynamics of the work of nursing?
4. Am I continually adjusting the role of nursing, i.e., creating and adapting, as an evolutionary process supporting the comprehensive health-care system?

Technical Competency Checklist

1. Are you able to manage complex multidisciplinary meeting processes and achieve desired goals?
2. Are your project management skills adequate?
3. Are employees/team members able to solve problems effectively?
4. Is decision making based on evidence?
5. Are customer needs and expectations managed?
6. Is there a succession plan in place?
7. What skills are you missing?

Interpersonal Competency Guidelines

1. Listen carefully to others.
2. Be fully engaged when others are speaking; do not think ahead or of other things.
3. Ask for feedback about your trustworthiness.
4. Ask for input and guidance, not only about new ideas but also about daily routines.
5. Request feedback regularly from those outside your normal group to determine how your work is impacting others.

Political Competency Guidelines

1. Be aware of the impact of the state board of nursing, Centers on Medicare/Medicaid Services, and the department of health services within your state on the practice of nursing.
2. Participate in organizations that impact the practice of nursing.
3. Expect colleagues to actively participate in nursing and health-care policy organizations.
4. Meet with your state legislator at least every three months.
5. Invite legislator to your organization to share ideas and influence policy.

Commercial Competence Guidelines

1. Seek out financial experts for the mechanics of accounting—you can't know it all.
2. Identify the economic value of nursing in the marketplace using evidence-based research.
3. Document cost-effectiveness of nurse interventions in your department/service/ organization.
4. Recognize the limitations of the current financing system and its impact on access to care.

Governance Competence Guidelines

1. Articulate one clear nursing vision for the organization—avoid the tendency to create a vision for every department.
2. Translate and review the mission, vision, and values for all employees at least annually.
3. Proactively evaluate the protection of patient rights—establish measures to demonstrate the rights are protected.

for their integrity, trust, respect, presence, and ability to form meaningful alliances. Further, diversity of thought, culture, and demographics are seen as essential to ensure that each person is able to contribute in unique and different ways for meaningful relationships.

Political competency is the dual capacity to accurately assess the impact of public policies on the performance of one's domains of responsibility and to influence public policy making at state, federal, and international levels. The nurse with political competency knows what the rules or policies are for the profession and the industry, knows who or what organization created them, the rationale for their existence, and how they impact the provision of health-care services. When an existing policy is identified as no longer appropriate or as negatively impacting health care, the nurse leader is both proactive and reactive in addressing the need for change.

One example is the multistate licensure of nurses. At one time, state-supported nurse licensure was appropriate. In the global world in which nurses are increasingly mobile, this model for licensure no longer protects the public as well as a multistate licensure model would. Thus, the politically competent nurse is knowledgeable of the policy of the state board of nursing, the rationale for the policy, and recommendations to change current policy to more appropriately support the provision of safe patient care. Nurses must be able to clearly state the impact of fiscal policy on health-care outcomes. Most importantly, the politically competent nurse is proactive about the issue rather than reticent to comment.

Commercial competence addresses the economic exchanges between buyers and sellers in which value is created. It is the knowledge and skill to establish and operate value-creating situations in which economic exchanges between patients/learners and the health-care system occur. The nurse with commercial competence is able to identify and provide care that makes a difference in patient outcomes within the boundaries of available resources. This competence is more than understanding basic cost accounting principles and the mechanics of developing a budget. The nurse with commercial competence understands reimbursement models as opportunities for nurses to demonstrate their unique contributions, understands the relationships among reductions in revenue, patient safety, quality outcomes, nurse satisfaction, and professional standards, and is able to use research to demonstrate which nursing interventions are consistent with cost-effective patient care. In essence, the nurse with commercial competence has the financial knowledge necessary to make decisions that integrate the clinical and business aspects of health care and value cost-effectiveness.

Governance competence addresses the establishment and enactment of a clear vision for the organization and includes the knowledge and skill to establish and enact the vision. Nurse leaders with expertise in governance competence are able to integrate the values of nursing within the organization and to create a culture that supports realization of the vision while providing care in the organization. Governance competence is about consistency among organizational values and beliefs, the tenets of the discipline of nursing, and the actual work of the organization. Examples of governance competence include ability to role model patient rights and welfare in decision making, formalization of nursing's vision, mission, and objectives, ensuring performance from nursing by establishing standards of care and a work setting that promotes quality care, and creation of a cultural system that allows teams to deliver patient care and hold professionals accountable for practice, work processes, teamwork, and outcomes.

Organizational Transparency vs. Overmanagement of Information

With the proliferation of management information systems, the amount and types of data generated are overwhelming. Leaders are expected to protect proprietary information and preserve the reputation of the organization. Leaders are also expected not to create roadblocks to information access when access to that information is appropriate. Creation of unnecessary roadblocks adds additional work for staff and frustrates those requesting the information. The ability to know the difference is an essential leadership competency. At times, health-care leaders have worked diligently to conceal information under the guise of protecting one's license, avoiding liability, and minimizing patient and family upsets. According to Kerfoot (2004), this concealment is at the heart of an organization's dysfunctional relationship among staff, patients, and families. Concealing information creates additional work processes that do not achieve the desired outcome and that cause employees to overanalyze information and wonder what is missing, creating a sense of caution and distrust.

Consumer Information

Openness or information transparency in organizations benefits the community, employees, and patients. Secrecy paralyzes learning, and performance cannot be improved without full disclosure (Berwick, 2004). As consumers become the directors of their own health care, openness with patients in health-care organizations is essential. Patients are indeed the best source of truth about their personal health and health-care professionals need to provide information they have gained to enhance the patient's ability to manage his or her own health care.

Caregiver Information

Consumers can easily access information on the Internet specific to appliances and vehicle safety. Similar information and resources must also be available from and accessed by health-care organizations and providers.

Caregivers should know the outcomes of their patient care process, what is being measured, how they compare to other units and similar units in other organizations, and what improvements are possible to continue the journey to excellence in patient care.

Organizational Information

Records of outcomes, satisfaction, and costs serve to assist consumers in making informed decisions. Access to this information becomes the accountability of the organization in order to assure that consumers not only know services and potential health-care interventions but also the level of performance of organizations that provide those services. Both the numbers of cases and outcomes should be readily available to current and potential consumers.

Differentiating confidential information from readily available and often public information requires knowledge of the owner of the information, regulatory requirements, and expected use of the information. Taking time to determine what really should be protected and what information is readily available to the public is important for minimizing the creation of unnecessary bureaucratic processes. Creating

Patient Care Unit Outcomes

1. Average number of patients/day; average length of stay
2. Patient satisfaction level
3. Number/type of medication errors
4. Number of patient falls
5. Number of urinary tract infections
6. Number of nosocomial pneumonia infections
7. Employee satisfaction level
8. Percentage of RNs/LPNs/NAs providing care
9. Cost of registry RNs
10. Average cost of care/day

a more trusting organization or organizational transparency should be the norm, rather than concealing information. Leaders need to be willing to share information that belongs to patients and to enter into meaningful dialogue to explain issues and decisions that are within their ability to disclose. This reinforces the value of trusting relationships. In contrast, leaders resistant to information sharing, fearful of dialogue in which patients will challenge the information, and belief that others will not understand the issues further reinforces a culture of secrecy and skepticism.

Rewards Without Evidence

Another source of toxicity is within the reward and recognition systems of an organization. Linking recognition and rewards to the desired competence and performance of caregivers continues to challenge the health-care industry. Multiple roles, multiple clinical settings, and multiple generational values provide a backdrop that does not support single or standardized reward and recognition programs. Yet, given this complexity, most organization offer standardized benefits and pay structures in the name of fairness and consistency. The emphasis in this mindset is on the *processes* of rewards and recognition rather than the desired outcomes of performance.

One of the most troubling practices is the annual awards banquets. Employees who have been physically present in the organization for numbers of years are recognized and rewarded in one of the most significant and costly events of the organization. This occurs in the face of organizational marketing touting clinical excellence, community involvement, and an environment of patient safety, none of which receives the level of reward and recognition of the annual employee attendance banquet. The challenge remains to recognize and reward employees who have contributed to the outcomes of quality patient care.

Nursing clinical ladders offer opportunities to transition from the traditional attendance reward system to one based on clinical competence and outcomes. The Nebraska Medical Center met the challenge of creating an effective management tool to recognize and reward clinical excellence by the creative use of consultants. The medical center identified the need to revise its clinical ladder to increase the credibility of the program and to ensure that rewards were linked to patient care outcomes and system goals. Using a nursing consultant and a human resource consultant as a team, goals were clarified, clinical excellence was redefined, and realistic financial incentives were created.

Key features of the program included:

- A specific annual dollar amount dedicated to the program
- An identified number of positions that would be available each quarter
- A clinical expert/nurse manager sponsor required, to assist the nurse in achieving the designation of clinical expert
- The majority of nurses recognized as proficient
- Level 2 of the program included nurses with national certification and a specific percentage salary increase
- Rewards for the expert status were segmented into 30% of the dollar amount for continuing education and 70% of the dollar amount in lump sum or other financial options
- Recognition of expert nurses as "Donors of Knowledge" along with other hospital donors identified with plaques in the main entrance

---

Rationale for The Nebraska Medical Center Clinical Ladder

- Recognition of clinical expertise is essential to retain clinical experts
- Responsible management of resources in anticipating and providing support for applicants is expected
- Responsible budget forecasting that begins with clear goals will assist in long-range planning
- Candidates will be supported to be successful!

Examples of Award Criteria for Excellence

1. Patient satisfaction scores above the norm
2. Development of innovative plans for individualized patient care
3. Resource to new and experienced nurses
4. Accountability for ongoing competence

Members of the clinical ladder program developed the following list of behaviors and competencies essential to the role of the expert. The unique feature of the program is the requirement for the presence of all competencies as described below. Nurses at the expert nurse level possess the competencies and must be able to provide evidence. Five categories of behaviors include:

1. *Clinical Excellence (Nurse Content).* The expert nurse is able to manage complex patients with multiple diagnoses, requiring multiple interventions. Managing family stress and customized patient education are examples of patient complexity. The nurse demonstrates clinical forethought, anticipation of patient needs and proactive planning, ability to assist patients and their families to manipulate/navigate the health-care system using complex critical thinking skills. Documents services accurately, concisely, and legibly.

2. *Patient Advocate.* The expert nurse promotes excellence through patient advocacy. The expert nurses questions inappropriate clinical actions, behaviors, and/or orders and initiates system changes to avoid repeat behaviors. The expert nurse challenges the system appropriately, i.e., in a timely manner and in a respectful manner. The expert nurse takes risks to modify the system rules to assure patient safety.

3. *Expert Resource.* The expert nurse serves as a confident and credible resource to others through the roles of: preceptor, which includes orientation to technical and relational behaviors of the organization; coach, which provides intermittent assistance with technical and relational behaviors and course corrects when appropriate; and mentor, which includes specific commitment to an individual for a designated time period. The expert nurse demonstrates and shares knowledge about the organization and the health-care environment.

4. *Role Model.* The expert nurse role models therapeutic behaviors, i.e., behaviors that improve the status of the individual following an interaction. The expert nurse is a team player and is viewed as a stress reducer rather than a stress producer. The expert nurse is able to refocus a stressed group of team members or patients/physicians. The expert nurse delegates duties to appropriate individuals and intervenes to ensure there is appropriate delegation.

5. *Accountability.* The expert nurse is able to demonstrate accountability for personal/professional development during the last three months. The expert nurse is knowledgeable about the changing practices of nursing and current health-care system processes.

The Magnet Bandwagon

The desire for recognition within the industry can become toxic when there is a disconnect between the infrastructure, goals, and processes to achieve those goals. The recognition and award should be the *result* of practice excellence, not the *driver* of the process just because others are doing it. Leaders may be able to envision the goals needed to achieve quality outcomes but cannot envision and create the appropriate supportive infrastructure with organizational processes and the desired goal. The endpoint of clinical excellence is recognized, while the processes of achieving the recognition are negated or not valued. It seems obvious to note that merely desiring an organization steeped in excellence is not enough and that the infrastructure, processes, values, and commitment

14 Forces of Magnetism
1. Quality of nursing leadership
2. Organizational structure
3. Management style
4. Personnel policies and programs
5. Professional models of care
6. Quality of care
7. Quality assurance
8. Consultation and resources
9. Level of autonomy
10. Community & the hospital
11. Nurses as teachers
12. Image of nursing
13. Collegial nurse-physician relationships
14. Professional development

to cultures of excellence must be present and in the right relationship, but it is necessary since are all essential components to achieve the goal of organizational excellence are too often not present or considered.

The Magnet bandwagon is one recent example. As many organizations achieve Magnet status recognition, the attractiveness of the recognition and attempt to get on the bandwagon is escalating. Some view Magnet recognition as merely a process to document current practices rather than evidence of organizational systems, processes, and outcomes that reflect the highest level of excellence in patient care and the organizational culture supportive of nursing. Even more problematic are the challenges to change Magnet standards to be more reflective of the current reality! Consider the efforts to modify the credentials of the chief nurse executive and allow nurse executives without a baccalaureate in nursing to be reflective of nursing excellence. While the nurse executive may have a bachelor's and master's degree in a health-related field, the lack of at least a bachelor's in nursing is inconsistent with excellence in nursing. Excellence in nursing leadership is about knowledge, relationships, effective processes, and achievement of exceptional outcomes—a comprehensive model rather than pieces.

Shared leadership is another example. Magnet standards include the expectation of shared leadership rather than autocratic models of decision making. Organizations declare shared leadership in their quest for Magnet status, then establish the traditional councils and continue to make decisions on the basis of individual role and position. The councils are merely window dressing for the survey process. The past is couched in the structure of new policies and language, but it is readily evident to members of the organization that past practices continue to be the norm. The Magnet journey is devalued to the Magnet bandwagon. Changing organizational structure and processes should be made to reflect the vision, mission, and intention of the organization, not the desire for a certain credential or award.

REVERSING TOXICITY: CREATING SUSTAINABLE SOLUTIONS

The work of healers is never finished. Removing negative influences and creating healing conditions is the essence of the healing leader. This work necessarily requires understanding the broad landscape of human behaviors and knowing which behaviors fit with one's personal and organizational vision and which behaviors cannot be tolerated if the healing journey is to continue. The challenge will always be to differentiate between the appropriate behaviors and inappropriate behaviors and to sustain and enhance the positive while isolating and minimizing the negative influences.

ONE MORE STRATEGY

Throughout this chapter strategies to reverse toxicity have been presented to assist the leader in creating healthy, healing cultures that will meet the need of patients, employees, and the community. The additional strategy of storytelling is presented to continue this journey.

Stories as Motivators

Most leaders are comfortable with the analytical process as a way of thinking to discover factual information, minimize myths, gossip, and speculate. The strength of the analytical process lies in its objectivity, its impersonality, and its heartlessness (Denning, 2004). Yet, to motivate individuals to live the vision and values of the organization with enthusiasm and energy, a more personal and heartwarming approach is needed to supplement the traditional PowerPoint presentations.

The age-old practice of storytelling can be one of the most effective tools of the leader. A story that has applicability to current practice and identifies both desired and undesired behaviors provides a method of teaching values that can achieve several goals.

Recently, a colleague was asked to present a keynote address to a health care audience. Knowing that the audience had heard it all about health care reform, the leader opted to tell a story of two experiences. Her address, "The state of healthcare?" did not have objectives, a beginning, or a well-developed middle, but it did have a thunderous ending. This story touched each person in the room in ways that were never anticipated, thus forever changing the practices of each person in the audience.

Storytelling Rationales
• Spark action
• Communicate who you are
• Transmit values
• Foster collaboration
• Tame the grapevine
• Share knowledge
• Lead people into the future
Stephen Denning, 2004

The story is as follows:

An elderly woman was admitted into the small-town hospital by her son and daughter-in-law for circulatory problems. Most caregivers knew the patient and worked to make her feel comfortable. The patient was evaluated and determined to need surgery. Unfortunately, the surgery could not be performed at the small hospital, so the patient was transferred to a large urban facility. The first night of patient's stay in the large facility was quite eventful. The patient was found out of bed in the middle of the night roaming the hall and was determined to be incoherent and subsequently restricted to bed. The patient begged for her son to be called, to no avail. The next day, nurses informed the family that a sitter was needed to assure the safety of the patient. In discussing the situation with the patient, it was learned that the patient needed to go to the bathroom and did not want to bother anyone; thus the confusion and subsequent restrictions. The next night the patient needed to go to the bathroom (at about the same time!) and attempted to get over the rails and blankets that were placed around her. Not surprisingly, the patient fell and fractured her hip. The speaker ended the story with, "So what's wrong with healthcare today—we're disconnected, over-automated, and can't get the basics of human elimination in the elderly managed, and my mother-in-law has a broken hip." The room was silent.

Such stories are all too common and provide insight and instruction to more issues than a textbook could. Using stories to make health-care services better can only help us be better healers.

SUMMARY

Most organizations are diligently working to meet deadlines, address national initiatives, achieve quality outcomes, and of course, make money. Unfortunately, many leaders get caught up in the busyness of their roles and the intended work of healing does not occur. Some very toxic practices and behaviors may emerge and undermine the hard work of all members of the organization.

This chapter offers new perspectives about the sources of toxicity, not to demoralize the leader but to offer insights that others have shared and strategies to correct negative processes. The realities of new employee hazing, destructive confidants, poor feedback, and working with those who just don't want to change should serve to motivate the quantum leader to assist all employees to be aware of these behaviors, call them to participate in minimizing the negative impact, and continue the quantum journey of leadership in the new age of technology.

Exercise 1 Partial Leadership

The description of the cardiovascular surgeon with exceptional technical skills, good patient outcomes and very poor interpersonal skills is a familiar to nurses. All too familiar also is the manager or leader with partial leadership skills—good negotiation skills, ability to develop a reasonable budget, and very poor performance evaluation skills due to the lack of ability to address conflict. Thus the overall reputation of the manager leader is less than stellar.

1. In your leadership group, discuss the differing skill levels of essential leadership behaviors. List the essential skills.
2. What skills are most often present?
3. What skills are often lacking? Develop a plan to address partial leadership.

Exercise 2 Removing the Barriers to Information

Technology now allows Internet access in each patient's room, wireless, real-time computerized documentation, integrated laboratory, medical imaging/diagnostic, and clinical progress. While these advances are relatively new and still being refined, the consumer now wants to be in charge of his or her data.

1. Given the availability of data and capabilities of the system, how would it be possible for patient information to go directly to the patient before or at the same time as the ordering provider receives the results?
2. For the patient to review and edit progress notes made about his or her care?
3. What expectations would need to be defined specific to the ordering of diagnostic tests?
4. What new skills would providers need to support these processes?
5. What security/access requirements would need to be in place to assure compliance with HIPPA?
6. What other issues need to be addressed?

REFERENCES

Berwick, D. (2004). *Escape fire: Designs for the future of health care.* San Francisco: Jossey Bass.

Carroll, V. (2003). Verbal abuse in the workplace: How to protect yourself and help solve the problem. *AJN* 103(3), 132.

Contu, D. L. (2003). I was greedy, too. *Harvard Business Review* 81(2), 38–44.

Cooper, R. W., Frank, G. L., Gouty, C. A., & Hansen, M. C. (2002). Key ethical issues encountered in healthcare organizations: Perceptions of nurse executives. *JONA* 32(6), 331–337.

Denning, S. (2004). Telling tales. *Harvard Business Review* 82(5), 122–129.

Goldsmith, J. (1998, July 5). Operation restore human values. *Hospitals & Health Networks,* 74.

Hofmann, P. B. (2004, March/April). Why good people behave badly. *Healthcare Executive,* 40.

Jackman, J. M., & Strober, M. H. (2003). Fear of feedback. *Harvard Business Review* 81(4), 101–107.

Kerfoot, K. (2004). On leadership: The transparent organization: Leadership in an open organization. *Nursing Economic$* 22(1), 33–34.

Longest, B. B. (1998). Managerial competence at senior levels of integrated delivery systems. *Journal of Healthcare Management* 43(2), 115–135.

Malloch, K. (2003). Leaders of the pack: Leadership model focuses on RN's authoritative role to boost uniformity, job satisfaction. *NurseWeek* 8(7), 9–10.

Mason, D. J. (2003). Tell me a story: Knowing when and how to use nursing stories. *AJN* 103(12), 7.

McMurry, R. N. (2003). The tyranny of groupthink. *Harvard Business Review* 81(7), 20.

McNulty, E. (2002). Welcome aboard (but don't change a thing). *Harvard Business Review* 80(2), 82–40.

Sulkowicz, K. J. (2004). Worse than enemies: The CEO's destructive confidant. *Harvard Business Review* 82(2), 65–71.

SUGGESTED READING

Lencioni, P. M. (2003). The trouble with teamwork. *Leader to Leader.* 29, 35–40.

The Leader as Mentor and Coach

CHAPTER OBJECTIVES:

Upon completion of this chapter, the reader will:

1. Clarify the need for a coach and mentor relationship and articulate its value in advancing leadership skills.

2. Describe the elements of coaching in the new age of leadership with emphasis on 21st-century leadership development.

3. Articulate the components of coaching and mentoring and apply them to the exercise of leadership at every level of the organization.

4. Identify the value of coaching and mentoring as a fundamental part of the management process and making it a part of the exercise of leadership.

INTRODUCTION

We're clearly entering a new age for leadership. New skills are not required in order for success in the exercise of the leader role. The 20th-century models for leadership rested primarily on the role of leader as a controlling agent. This notion of control and gender-driven management incorporates a whole range of skills that were essentially parental in nature and hierarchical in expression. This understanding of leadership as a hierarchical, controlling role drove much of the competency and content of the leadership role during the whole of the 20th century.

The problem with a controlling and hierarchical leadership is reflected specifically in its role expectations and performance requirements. In exercising the role of the leader in a hierarchical organization, there is a need on the part of the organization for the leader to represent the best interests of the organization and to see to it that workers' efforts are directed to the organization's goals. As a result, the leader's role historically has been focused on assuring that the organization's goals were met consistently and with the level of expectations the organization had for the work. The role of the leader was primarily expressed in the functions and activities related to supervising and controlling workers' actions and activities. It was assumed that the followers needed constant attention

The Role of the Industrial–Age Leader
Planning
Organizing
Leading
Controlling
Evaluating

and supervision in order to do their work well. The leader was primarily required to act as a "parent," and the organization assumed that in this role the leader would ensure that the workers (the children) of the organization did as they should or, at least, as they were directed. The organization represented the belief that workers would not meet its goals or fulfill its requirements if they did not have appropriate supervision and direction, provided by a "good" leader. This notion of directing the activities of others gave the leader role authority and responsibility for ensuring that work was appropriately done. Certain assumptions regarding the leader's skills and abilities were made under the rubric of supervision. It was assumed that the leader had the same knowledge about the work as the workers did and that the subordinate's level of knowledge and the leader's positional authority ostensibly gave the leader greater skill and deeper understanding of the work than those who had actually performed it. The authority for work outcomes was essentially invested in the exercise of the leadership role rather than in the performance of the work role.

The control function in the organization predominantly defined the managerial role. The expectation of the leader was that the department or service was well run, orderly, controlled, and disciplined, quietly and efficiently achieving predetermined outcomes. Essentially, the workforce was to see to it that the work was done, and the leader's job was to ensure that happened. Disciplining the workforce and keeping workers focused on the work were the requisites of leadership, as was doing so with a minimum level of "noise." Leaders who were successful in running their departments or services kept the staff noise level down, minimized the acting-out of problem workers, and reduced the number of worker problems, thus enhancing productivity and assuring that the organization's outcomes were met. The notion of *control* drove the value of excellence and performance within the context of the role of the leader.

Of course, this contextual framework for the role of the leader was not sustainable. In organizations today, it is recognized that adult-to-adult relationships are essential to organizational effectiveness. They replace notions of parent-child models of leadership and relationship. Current research shows that these new leadership models that reflect partnership, interaction, and adult behaviors actually facilitate work, as opposed to the controlling models, which were more of an impediment to effective work than an assist to it.

Leaders are predominantly context creators. In creating an appropriate context, the leader builds a frame of reference within which the organization can operate. This context either creates opportunities for meaningful work and positive relationships or draws away from the environment necessary to do good work and to achieve meaningful outcomes. The leader understands the relationships necessary to produce positive outcomes and maintain a meaningful work environment. The leader also recognizes that all people are social creatures and thus reflects the understanding of the necessity of good social interaction and positive relationships in order to maintain high levels of productivity. The challenge is that the leader must recognize that workers are essentially partners who must establish collaborative and meaningful relationships in order to sustain productivity and to enhance the work of the organization.

As with all relationships, the leader recognizes that interaction must go through a number of stages, each of which must be thoroughly addressed, in order to ensure the highest levels of integrity and work quality. In this set of circumstances, the leader is primarily a coach working in a framework that fully enables individuals to be successful. The leader knows that encouraging and strengthening the relationships between

The 20th-Century Leader Expectations

- Keep workers focused on the "job"
- Make sure workers were not "noisy"
- Ensure work is focused and detailed
- Keep workers "happy"
- Discipline workers appropriately
- Resolve inevitable worker conflicts
- Supervise workers closely
- Be specifically directive with clear expectations
- See that the work is done well

Controlling vs. Engaging Leadership

Controlling	Engaging
• hierarchical	• equitable
• assumes superiority	• role-based
• directive style	• inclusive
• highly positional	• reflects parity
• detailed supervision	• horizontal dialogue
• criticism-based	• exploratory

Different Expectations for Communication

Adult-to-adult	Parent-child
• respect-based	• safety-based
• acknowledges unique talents	• developmental
• inclusive	• instructive
• reflects equity	• reflects superiority
• eliminates hierarchy	• vertical dialogue
• open and free-flowing	• directed and clear

leader and workers and between workers creates circumstances and a context that assures meaningful, purposeful, and energy-filled activity directed to fulfilling the purposes and goals of the organization.

COACHING AND EXPECTATIONS

The leader must reflect in his or her coaching role an understanding of performance expectations and others' related behavior. The leader is always aware that performance is an integral part of the fulfillment of the demands of work. Furthermore, relationships demand a clear understanding of what people expect from leaders. The leader does not leave role expectation to accident.

The wise leader establishes a framework for expectations. In fact, this leader contracts for expectations so the roles, functions, and activities performed by individuals either in a team or in relationship to the leader are clear and understandable in advance of establishing the relationship. When coaching is discussed, it is often exemplified in relationship to a one-on-one interaction. In truth, coaching relates to the individual as leader and to the leadership of groups. No leader simply establishes a relationship with one individual and then focuses solely on that person to exclusion of the relationship with all others. Coaching involves the collective relationship between all those with whom the leader interacts. The leader exemplifies in her or his behavior the expectations for performance and for the relationships that the leader seeks to see in others.

The greatest concern in most organizations is the conflicts that are often generated, problems associated with relationships and interactions between individuals. This focus on facilitating positive interaction frequently becomes the major focus of the leader's work. These behaviors and interactions are continually influenced by the ebb and flow of the group members' interaction and communication with each other. The leader attempts to build as positive a framework for these interactions as is possible and attempts to identify conflicts or impediments to smooth functioning relationships between and among team members.

The leader is always concerned with the interaction of the team. In the coaching role, the leader attempts to represent in her or his own behavior best practices in terms of expression, communication, interaction, and problem solving. Here, the leader is most interested in ensuring that a model of sound leader behavior is created and exemplifies this "model of behavior" in her or his own conduct. The challenge here is the consistency and continuity of the behavior in the message of the leader as coach. In this role, the leader clearly presents an example or set of behaviors that potentially can be exemplified in the expectations of the conduct of others. The leader is attempting through this behavior to create a model of expression and interaction that others can replicate in their own behavior.

THE LEADER IS ALWAYS "ON"

The leader is never "off." The leader's expectation is that all behaviors will be consistent and will be sustained. In this way, others can incorporate new patterns of leader behavior in their own roles because they witness good leader behavior as consistent and congruent. The leader becomes a living witness to the expectations of interaction, performance, and role behavior that serves as a model for each member of the work team.

> ### Gem
>
> Coaching relates to all the relationships of leadership. The coach recognizes that all relationships serve as a potential for ideal behaviors and commitment to growth. The coach is available to all through the representation of the role as an exemplar. The coach models the role so that all people are informed by it and seek to include the ideal behaviors in their own practices and roles.

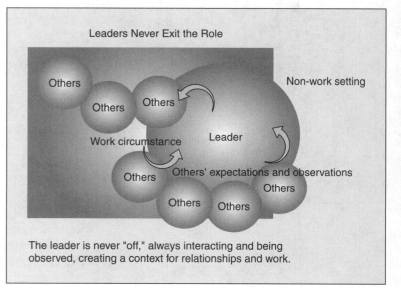

The leader is never "off," always interacting and being observed, creating a context for relationships and work.

The Coaching Contract Basics

- The contract is voluntary
- Language is specific and clear
- The leader lives the elements of the agreement
- Contract can be adjusted as reality requires

CONTRACTING FOR EXPECTATIONS

A contract for expectations is simply a delineation of those performance factors that must be most often considered and exemplified in the role of each team member. This contract is entered into as an agreement between all members of the team and with the leader. In this contract, there are specific elements that are critical to the expression of expectations and commitments made by team members to each other:

1. The leader is clear at the outset that the contract is voluntary, underscores mutual expectations and behavioral determinations, is clearly an agreement to behave in a particular way, and is understood and excepted by all members of the team.
2. The contract is specific and clear. It is not left for team members to guess the expectations and performance factors that they must exemplify in their relationship with each other.
3. The leader agrees to not only abide by the charter and the commitment made by team members but to exemplify those behaviors in his or her own role. The team leader exemplifies membership and collaboration with team members by virtue of her or his own collaborative and interactional role characteristics.
4. The team commitments or charter is not cast in stone, as behavioral expectations and patterns of relationship will shift. Change in the content of the charter should also reflect a mutual understanding of the commitment of all parties. Each shift in expectations and performance factors should be included in the charter, reflecting it as a living document. As this contract moves and shifts in content, it can be redesigned to reflect the new expectations and different patterns of behavior.

Not all contracts have to be written agreements. The notion of contracting reflects an understanding between the team members and the leader regarding certain sets of behaviors and expectations that they have agreed to between and among themselves. Written documentation of these processes simply acts as a certification or verification that these agreements have been entered into. Whether or not the contract is written down, all parties to the contract assume some responsibility for ensuring that their behaviors will be consistent with their agreement and with the expectations for performance.

Accountability with regard to performance requires that individuals be willing to commit to reviewing and evaluating each other with regard to certain expectations. The leader clearly must be aware that these evaluation processes are fraught with general difficulties and much noise. When one is evaluating another individual, there are a number of sensitivities that emerge that must be addressed carefully and thoughtfully if such evaluation is not to degenerate into untenable and unacceptable critique. This requires that some measure of performance expectation and evaluation be discussed and clarified before performance evaluation occurs. Each member of the team, building the expectations for other members of the team, must be clear about how to approach and interact with others during evaluation of an individual's performance or behavioral pattern. The challenge for the leader is to exemplify good

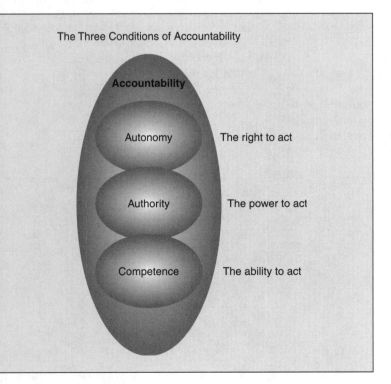

The Three Conditions of Accountability

Accountability

Autonomy — The right to act

Authority — The power to act

Competence — The ability to act

communication and conflict management patterns in her or his own behavior so that these patterns can be reflected in the behaviors of those he or she leads. In a coaching situation, team members will be looking critically at the role of the leader as that person undertakes the active evaluation of another, assessing performance or adjusting behavior.

Again, the leader's role is to exemplify desired behaviors in the leader's own behavior. Perhaps this is the central heart of all mentoring and coaching relationships. Staff is continually observing leaders and learning what their consistency is in terms of their own behavior and just what the vagaries of that behavior is. The leader must know that every moment she or he is being observed within the context of the leadership role.

It is often said that leaders have no friends. This is especially true in a coaching and mentoring situation. Yet it's surprising how many leaders forget that leadership is a particular role, one in which friendship is not an element. The mentor and coach leader must always recall the role that he or she plays in relationship to those being mentored or coached. The relationship between leader and those being coached has a particular set of structures and characteristics that is unique to it. The leader recognizes this reality and does not attempt to confuse those he or she is coaching by exemplifying other kinds of relationships not appropriate to the role. The notion of always being "in role" is a critical part of understanding the role of the leader, especially in the process of mentoring and coaching. Leading implies setting direction and moving others to embrace the journey and to incorporate it into their own experiences and lives. The coach and mentor helps others engage their own reality, identify their own role in relationship to it, and embrace the activities and functions necessary to achieve it. This is done by the leader exemplifying the degree of commitment and by embracing and engaging the dynamics of change and the demands of the role in the life of the leader. Using this living example as the frame of reference for coaching and mentoring becomes the most viable tool the leader has to advance and incorporate appropriate and desirable behaviors in others, especially in regard to interaction, relationship, and embracing the future.

Contracted factors in coaching agreement

Expectations · Roles · Communication · Evaluation factors & timeline

Coach's Role
Define expectations, roles, measures, rules of engagement, conditions of coaching relationship

Coaching Performance Assessment Factors

Gem

Friendship is not a component of the leadership role. In short, leaders have no friends. The leader is entering risky territory if friendships impact the exercise of the leadership role. The leader is always "in role" when expressing and experiencing leadership within the organization. Leaders must never forget that they are continually being observed by staff within the context of their role. Therefore, leaders should always be acting in the role—failing to do so creates confusion and ultimately loss of respect for the role.

DEMONSTRATING GOOD DECISION MAKING

Besides exemplifying good behaviors, interactions, and collaborative relationships, the leader must exemplify the skills of good decision making. The leader's application of the skills and ability to develop and expand decision-making talent becomes a foundational skill set for those the leader coaches and mentors. There is, perhaps, no other skill more important to the development of leadership than the ability to make effective decisions.

Decision making is not an accidental process. Decisions are not effective simply because people make them. Good decisions require insight, creativity, and methodology. The good leader recognizes and understands that if good decision making is to be replicated it must involve a process that is organized

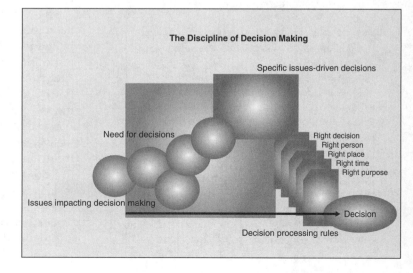

The Discipline of Decision Making

Specific issues-driven decisions

Need for decisions

Right decision
Right person
Right place
Right time
Right purpose

Issues impacting decision making

Decision

Decision processing rules

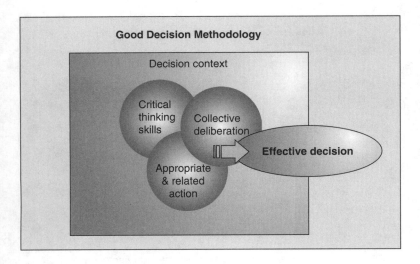

Good Decision Methodology

Decision context

Critical thinking skills

Collective deliberation

Appropriate & related action

Effective decision

Maximizing Information Sources

- Review what is at hand
- Determine what can be readily accessible
- Use Internet sources
- Access readily available historic data
- Have conversations with key stakeholders
- Speak with colleagues who have previous experience
- Sort the relevant from the merely interesting
- Focus information within defined time frame
- Select information based on priority of impact

Evaluating Good Decision Making

- Did the decision relate directly to the problem?
- Was the desired outcome achieved?
- What information was helpful in arriving at the decision?
- What was the relationship between the information, the decision, and the outcome?
- What information was most helpful?
- What information was of least value?
- How do others perceive the decision and its outcome?
- What would you do differently next time?
- What information was missing?
- What process barriers did you confront?
- What learning did this decision and its outcome provide for you?
- How will you proceed differently next time?

---

and systematic and can be replicated. In working with the team, the leader represents in her or his own behavior a specific discipline or set of processes within which decision making unfolds. *The leader does not make decisions for others.* Instead, the leader positions other individuals to make decisions by ensuring that the appropriate decisions, skills, and patterns of decisional behavior are incorporated into the role of that person that he or she mentors.

There are essential characteristics to effective decision making. Good decision makers always understand that there is a discipline to decision making, as there is to any other organized work activity. Good decision making involves a number of process steps to ensure that the decision will be effective and produce the desired results:

1. *The use of good methodology.* A leader recognizes that decisions have components and elements expressed in stages. When articulated and defined clearly enough, these processes can be followed and replicated in all decision processes. The leader recognizes that critical thinking, deliberation, and responsive action all work together to create a framework for the effective application of decision making. Building a clear methodology is an essential cornerstone for effective decision making, regardless of who is involved.

2. *Gathering information.* All good decisions are made with as much information as possible under the circumstances. What is important to remember is that no one has all the information needed to make effective decisions. The point is not to have every bit of information that is available, but instead, to have sufficient information to make the right decision with the resources available at the time of decision making. The leader recognizes that decision making must be well informed to the extent possible at the needed time and recognizes that a lack of information is a part of the process. Therefore, the leader takes whatever information is available, aggregates it with other sources of information, synthesizes it, and decides the best course of action to take under the circumstances. Recognizing and managing limited information resources is not only good information management, it is good leadership.

3. *Good critical thinking skills.* Nothing replaces the ability to think clearly, logically, and appropriately at the right time and arrive at the right answer. Critical thinking reflects the ability of the individual to organize thought and to make decisions based on the integrated relationship of ideas, information management, and good response in a way that most effectively meets the demand of the situation or circumstance. Decision making simply is the result of having carefully considered all the elements related to and affecting a decision and proceeding with action followed by evaluation.

4. *Effective evaluation of decisions.* The leader always assesses the effectiveness of decision making in a meaningful way. A good mentoring and coaching technique is to involve others in evaluating an individual's decision making. The competent and balanced leader is not afraid of an evaluation of his or her own decision making because this helps clarify, refine, and improve that skill, both in the leader as well as in the mentor. In fact, the leader usually develops a formalized evaluation process so that evaluation is not simply a periodic and perhaps optional undertaking; it is, instead, a struc-

tured routine that is incorporated into the fundamental activity of decision making and of evaluation.

5. *Good error assessment processes.* The leader is not afraid of error. In fact, error is understood as a fundamental part of the experience of deliberation and decision making. No matter how effective the decision maker is, there will always be an element of error embedded in every decision and action. Ineffective decision making is not the greatest problem with regard to leadership. But the ability to successfully and effectively address errors at the right time and in the right format is essential. Error is not an untenable part of the activities of human life. The good mentor and coach demonstrates the ability to engage his or her own experience of error as part of the evaluation and deliberation process. The leader can mentor staff and coach new behaviors through exemplifying his or her own ability to self-evaluate and make critical judgments about the decision. The leader adjusts or changes patterns of behavior based on what the evidence reveals about the process, methodology, or outcomes of decision making. In this way, the leader demonstrates that error is not a source of fear or punishment; instead, it is an opportunity to learn, engage, and adjust performance and behavior based on what the evidence reveals.

6. *Creating effective corrective action processes.* Recognizing the inevitability of error, the leader incorporates that understanding into the process of responding to error. The leader indicates this through an organized and systematic corrective action process, demonstrating to those he or she is coaching or mentoring the engagement of corrective action as a normative and functional part of critical decision making. All decisions require assessment. Out of this assessment comes the need for a change in practices, behavior, or processes. The leader demonstrates the ease of incorporating the need for new practices and behaviors as a result of evaluating past practices and behaviors. Incorporating this understanding into leadership practices demonstrates for those being mentored and coached the desirability of evaluating of decision activities, the value of applying a critical method to evaluation processes, and the growth and development that results in the individual from undertaking this discipline. Error is thus transformed from a negative aspect of decision making to a positive part of the cycle of decision making. Error can become a fundamental part of the entire decision process and serve a critical role in helping to develop the decisional effectiveness of individuals and the excellent application and ultimate productivity of error management in the course of decision making and in advancing the quality of work.

IDENTIFYING COACHING GOALS

Coaching focuses on the needs of the person being coached. A part of establishing these needs is identifying the goals and specific objectives that the individual seeks to address through the coaching process. The goals initially are negotiated and agreed to by the coach and the person being mentored. Ultimately, however, the goals and specific objectives of the individual being coached must be owned and exercised by that individual. The individual looks to the coach for support and encouragement, as well as indicators and patterns of behavior that can be replicated and developed. Individuals are responsible for their own development and growth. It is the goal of the coach to make those being coached as independent as possible, needing as little coaching as possible. In fact,

---

Gem

Error is not a source of fear or punishment. Error a simply an opportunity for learning. The only errors that are unforgivable are those that are repeated. The continual repetition of the same error is a sign that little has been learned from it and that the participants in the error are doomed to continuously repeat it. Error is to be celebrated, acknowledged for its contribution to learning, and responded to appropriately and in a timely fashion. Doing so gives error its proper place and assures its role as a teacher bearing renewable fruits.

Corrective Action Processing

1. Locating the critical event (error)
2. Enumerating again the characteristics of an error
3. Identifying the learning embedded in the error
4. Naming the impact of the error
5. Discovering the source or foundation of the error
6. Delineating the process elements leading to the error
7. Listing effective corrective steps
8. Defining evaluation of corrective steps
9. Clarifying corrective steps and successful actions
10. Celebrating and sustaining newly defined behaviors

The Coaching and Mentoring Relationship

- Short term
- Goal-driven
- Owned by the person being coached
- Centered on learning
- Developmentally focused
- Performance-based
- Contains elements of evaluation
- Peer-based
- Ends when goals are completed

the primary role of the coach is to ensure that the individual being mentored has no extended need for the mentor and has developed sufficient skills to be able to act independently. In the coaching and mentoring relationship, the ultimate sign of success is when those being coached and mentored themselves become coaches and mentors to others. It is this goal of obtaining independence and being able to operate at the same level of facility or skill as the coach that becomes one of the primary operating criteria for a good coach-mentor relationship. The coach is always aware that the coaching relationship is short term. The coach does everything possible to ensure the growth and development of the individual being coached, to the extent that the individual will no longer need the same developmental processes and activities as at the beginning of the coaching-mentoring relationship.

When the coaching and mentoring goals are clearly defined and the expectations and performance against those goals unfolds, as they should, the coaching and mentoring relationship becomes developmental. As the developmental process unfolds and the individual being coached becomes more successful in their own patterns of behavior, two things occur. One key element is that the coaching relationship changes in form and substance as the individual matures and becomes increasingly independent. The second critical factor is that the coaching role transitions into a collaborative partnership role that continues the dynamic of relationship but simply changes the form in which it is expressed. It is in this relationship that the most significant value is obtained from the coaching-mentoring interaction. This relationship is one that can best delineate for those being coached a very specific valuing of purpose, achieving the highest level of outcome from the process.

A NEW AGE FOR LEADERSHIP

Leadership is unfolding in a time of great change. Mentoring and coaching means bringing people into a new era of leadership that requires different skill sets and roles. This evolution in organizational forms matches a significant change in the social culture and the global community. A part of the challenge for leaders is recognizing that the leader is now leading movements to new age. This notion of leading movement is critical to understanding the role of the leader and the changes in the expectation and performance of leadership.

Movement into the global community means a change in all organizational constructs. Furthermore, it means a change in the kinds of relationships and interactions that must unfold in order for organizations and systems to be successful. The challenge for the leader is having the ability to identify in her or his own behavior the kinds of role changes necessary to lead an organization into a quickly evolving world. Further complicating this challenge is the requisite that the leader be able to change her or his own behavior in a way that represents or characterizes a new set of expectations for expressing the role of leader. Being able to translate the skills sets necessary to lead in a new age and adapt those skill sets to a new model of organization is another critical exemplar for the role of leader as coach and mentor.

The mentor and coach now must incorporate in his or her own leadership behaviors mechanisms for building partnership, constructing alliances, defining new directions and constructs for the organization, negotiation and conflict resolution, and the management of complex systems and relationships. Each of these skill sets brings with it a specific set of demands that alters the leader's expectations and performance obligations.

The Coaching-Mentoring Partnership

- Is equity based
- Represents a set of defined expectations
- Roles are negotiated
- Evaluation of effectiveness is continuous
- There is a regularly scheduled dialogue
- The coach identifies other collaborators
- Team review is included
- Time expectations are clarified
- Relationship outcomes are clearly defined
- Performance expectations are regularly reviewed

Managing Movement

Leaders do not manage people. People manage themselves. The role of the leader is to create a safe context where people can adjust their patterns of work behavior to fit an ever-shifting context. The leader recognizes the movement of change, translates it in a language the follower can comprehend, and finally enables the follower to fully engage the changes affecting the dynamic of work in a way that can continue to produce positive and meaningful outcomes.

Organization around team-based approaches requires a different kind of facility with regard to leadership. Hierarchical relationships often defined the past, traditional approach to leadership. Now, because systems are membership communities, the leader must exemplify a different set of more horizontally aligned behaviors. The leader must form partnerships and alliances in an effective array of interactions and intersections that help organizations move in concert toward the goals necessary to thrive. The challenge in a complex world is the balance between competition and cooperation. Leaders must exemplify for those they are coaching and mentoring that neither competition nor cooperation are unilaterally effective in undertaking or advancing the organization's work. The leader must exemplify in his or her own behavior those times when cooperation predominates within the system, perhaps even with competitors. On the other hand, the leader also must exemplify those times when competition is necessary in order to advance the viability and success of the organization.

At the same time as the leader is handling concerns regarding competition and cooperation, ethical and relational issues emerge as increasingly important concerns. With communication and technical advances in systems processes affecting the work itself, a new sensitivity to the importance of ethics as incorporated into relationships, business practices, and corporate and organizational intersections emerges as a critical element of new leadership. The leader must exemplify in his or her own behavior those skills necessary to delineate the moral and ethical elements of relational, decisional, or operational issues. This has become increasingly evident in the current business environment. The leader must represent to the person being mentored or coached the moral and value implications in all processes of decision making. The leader must also represent that these behaviors must be incorporated into the activities necessary to positively express sound leadership in any circumstance. Decision making and effective decision processes should include the ethical and moral implications as a part of the planned process of effective decision making. Furthermore, mentors and those being coached should themselves exemplify the incorporation and evaluation of these patterns and practices of ethical and moral behavior in all decisions and actions.

DEVELOPING NEW ERA LEADERSHIP COMPETENCIES

In this new era of changing organizational forms and structures, leaders will require a certain level of entrepreneurial freedom as well as a set of self-directed skills that exemplify a new kind of engagement with the organization and its journey into a preferred future. In the industrial age, the leader represented for those learning new leadership skills a stronger orientation to function, effectiveness, and process. Although these elements are certainly important, they are no longer the centerpiece of work or the role of the leader. In the development of leadership in others, the leader must exemplify within the role a deeper understanding of its relationship to an organization's or system's journey and a willingness to perceive the response to that journey within the context of a larger social construct.

In a mentoring and coaching model, the leader must exemplify the notion of managing movement in a way that characterizes the pace and the direction of change for the organization. The leader sees the role within a much longer and larger trajectory. Using approaches that take into account the changing circumstances, conditions, innovations, and social

---

Using Competition vs. Cooperation for Obtaining Goals

Competition

- creating opposing forces
- generating energy in opposition
- beating others toward a target
- harnessing internal resources
- focusing action externally
- identifying a common foe

Cooperation

- creating converging forces
- enjoining group energy
- consolidating around common goal
- gathering all relevant resources
- focusing energy on group's efforts
- surpassing group's own standards

Questions of Ethical and Moral Leadership

- Is our position or initiatives consistent with our corporate values?
- Is our position or initiative legal?
- Does our position or initiative reflect defined standards of practice?
- Does our position or initiative violate any cultural norms?
- Are individuals purposely disadvantaged or harmed by our position or initiative?
- Do our efforts reflect sound business practices?
- Would our organization be ashamed if our efforts were made public?
- Do we have a mechanism for auditing and evaluating our work processes?
- Will the outcomes of our efforts have a negative social or environmental impact?
- Do our efforts raise our standard of performance and enhance the organization's image?

Entrepreneurial Leader Characteristics

- creatively individualistic
- is a self-starter
- sees things "out-of-the-box"
- has a powerful personal charisma
- is idea-driven
- explores all avenues
- engages others in creative work
- can move ideas to goals

Managing Movement

The contemporary leader understands that managing movement means helping people engage the challenges of their own journey. This leader recognizes that the failure of individuals to embrace the demands of their own personal change and to join that with the inevitable changes in work performance and expectation is most problematic. Leaders recognize that they exemplify willingness in their own behaviors and through personal example model agreement and engagement to continuously embrace every movement in the dance of change.

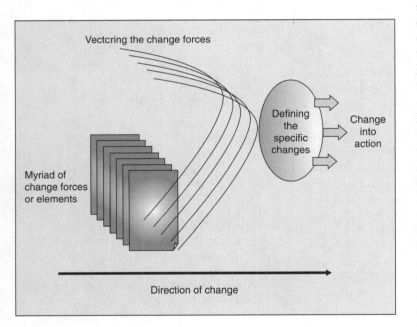

Deep Change

Real and sustainable change cannot occur unless there's a strong personal commitment on the part of the individual to undergo significant personal change. All of the mentoring in the world will not achieve successful outcomes if individual personal commitment is not present. In the mentoring and coaching process, the individual agrees to engage many challenges and vagaries associated with learning and growing and consents to not pull back from the demands of change when they become uncomfortable and raise potential personal difficulties.

challenges, the innovative leader undertakes appropriate responses configured to position the organization well within the context of its continuing journey. This fluidity and flexibility in approaches and response will be a critical foundational element if the leader is to influence and exemplify learning flexibility when both mentoring and coaching new leaders.

The leader exemplifies the skills of anticipation as a part of the development of sound leadership practices. The leader's talent for reading the signposts is an important transformational characteristic for coaching and mentoring. Reading signposts means taking the various factors that indicate imminent shift or changes at the sociological or organizational level and applying them to the unique work circumstances for which the leader is accountable. In this way, the leader "reads" the conditions, circumstances, and indicators that tell the story of the organization's journey in a way that anticipates the next steps. Through this leadership strategy of vectoring or signpost reading, the leader represents a willingness to engage the foundations of change and to bring form and substance to the direction of the change. It is this notion of bringing congruence between the direction of change and the response to the demand of change that most influences the appropriate development of leadership skills in others around the notion of harnessing talent for the future.

Here again, it is important to emphasize that the leadership coach and mentor doesn't underestimate the traditional values and role competencies related to cost effectiveness, organizational congruency, human relationship skills, decision making, and conflict resolution. What happens instead is that the leader also represents additional sets of behaviors that represent the changing context for leadership. The industrial age clearly had a more institutional, structured, and functional frame for the expression of leadership. In the sociotechnical age, contemporary roles of the leader are dramatically shifting to reflect the new characteristics of high technology, global communication, and fluidity and flexibility of work systems and organizational pursuits. This fundamental change in the notion of work and its exercise causes the coach and mentor to change the content and the frame for leading others and modeling that leadership for the future. Coaching and mentoring now becomes a set of challenges that helps individuals alter their frames of reference for leadership and form a new foundation for understanding and exercising the role as they learn it.

DEEP CHANGE: NEW WAYS OF BEING AND DOING

Thus far, the focus has been on the elements and constituents of coaching and mentoring the emerging leader into a new set of leader behaviors. Equally important is the commitment of the individual being coached or mentored to his or her own deep personal change. While leadership is clearly an important area of discussion and certainly a critical pursuit in the changing workplace, what is equally important is the need to understand that new leaders must represent an entirely different foundation for behavior. The coach must exemplify within the role a clear commitment to personal change through her or his own efforts and activities. Subsequent to any real change occurring, the people being mentored and coached must also evidence their own commitment to the "noise" of deep personal change.

This understanding of deep personal change goes further than a simple understanding of the change process. Deep personal change means adaptability and willingness to change. The person being coached or mentored needs to be able to express a willingness to undergo the challenges of change. This individual must greet a new paradigm for practice that incorporates the notion of managing continuous and endless movement and transformation within the context of individual personhood, as well as within the framework of the organization.

For the leader who is coach and mentor, exemplifying this behavior is a critical exemplar for the expression of good leadership. Leaders must always remember that they are constantly being watched by those they lead. The exemplar is the leaders' commitment to never forget their own behavioral patterns and the impact those patterns have on the skills and practices of others. This notion of willingness to embrace the reality of constant change and to engage it in a meaningful way using the skills identified here is the critical subtext for coaching and mentoring others.

COACHING FOR DEEP CHANGE

Change leaders and coaches must help those they are mentoring to recognize that leadership now is different in its expression and application than it was in the past. The move out of the industrial age is calling leaders to see their role differently as the context for leadership shifts. The challenges that emerge in the new age relate to the introduction of new technologies, global communication technologies, digitalization of information, and the application of new work processes to health care. In this shifting context, the coach represents in her or his own behavior a willingness to address what these challenges mean and how they call for a change in leadership behavior.

The coach must articulate for the learning leader a completely new frame of leadership skills. The primary role of the leader in today's world is to help others make the transition in their own practice and behavior to represent a much more fluid and mobile work environment. The coach exemplifies in willingness to meet the challenge related to unfolding the new framework for work and new work processes. Because of this, the coach begins to challenge the learning leader to see the role in a different light and to begin to articulate those skills that will be necessary to facilitate the changing role and work of others.

The coach seeks in the learning leader an ability to facilitate adaptation and to crystallize within the role positive behaviors that model willingness, availability, vulnerability, and a fundamental agreement to change the nature of work and the experience of the worker. The coach challenges the new leader to see the expression of leadership in light of the journey that the learning leader is experiencing as though he or she were already playing the leader role.

The new age requires a different contextual framework for the leader's role expression, from industrial-age direction and controlling mechanisms to the new expectations of leadership to engage relationships, communication, and skill transformation. In leading others (especially emerging leaders) to express their role in a transforming work environment, the coach challenges them to incorporate within the context of

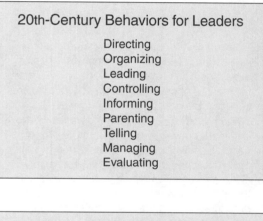

Modeling Change

Leaders cannot expect that those they mentor will make changes that leaders themselves will not undertake. Mentoring is essentially role modeling: exemplifying in one's own behavior those same behaviors one expects to see exemplified in those one mentors. Leadership is a lived circumstance that requires leaders to give evidence of having embraced specific changes in their own roles before asking others to change. Leaders cannot ask change in others that they have not undertaken in themselves.

20th-Century Behaviors for Leaders

Directing
Organizing
Leading
Controlling
Informing
Parenting
Telling
Managing
Evaluating

21st-Century Behaviors for Leaders

Clearinghouse
Enrolling
Investing
Conflicting
Challenging
Moderating
Inquiring
Facilitating
Stretching

Emerging New Leader Roles

Extinguishing "old" roles ———▶ Emerging "new" roles
Direction of change

• Directing
• Control
• Parenting
• Correcting

New Leader Role

• Coordinating
• Facilitating
• Gathering
• Integrating

Leadership Vulnerability

- an openness to discuss personal pain
- sharing insights regarding personal journey of change
- being clear about what is not known
- intuition regarding others' struggles
- willing to name one's personal difficulties with change
- gathering advice and counsel from others
- willing to explore all options
- good at information gathering and sharing
- unafraid of confronting difficulties/barriers
- recognizes the need and timing for self-renewal

Having the Right Questions

Traditionally the role of the manager/leader was tied to having the right answers to others' questions. The contemporary leader and mentor, instead of having the right answers, makes sure that the right questions are raised. Without the right question any answer will do. The leader never takes accountability for other people's answers. In order to assure that doesn't happen, the leader makes sure that ownership of the question is established and that those being mentored are focusing on the right questions instead of simply looking for the appropriate answer. Without the right question there is no right answer.

Creating a Safe Space

- People feel free to express their own concerns
- No retribution results from self-expression
- A context for problem-solving is present
- Adult-to-adult exchange is encouraged
- There are no undiscussables
- Conflicts are addressed quickly
- Dialogue and problem-solving is encouraged
- Fear-based language is stamped out early
- Negativity is never tolerated
- Hope and encouragement are expected of everyone
- Social interaction and humor is encouraged

their own behavior a facility at exploration, coaching, dialogue, and experimentation in the arena of new practices and processes. The learning leader also incorporates into her or his behavior an ability to engage others in conflict, respond to the noise of change, and deal effectively with the pace of change.

The coach's role in encouraging deep change includes being able to engage others at a personal level. First, the coach must exemplify in her or his own role an understanding of the impact of change on the self. This notion of understanding one's own accommodation or challenge with regard to the impact of change is an important prototype for providing an opportunity for the coach to role model that response for others. As the coach confronts personal inadequacy and represents that challenge in the coach's own transition to change, she or he begins to represent to those learning leaders her or his role modeling for change and how adjustments and accommodation to the challenges can be well addressed. If the coach is unable to accommodate change, face the noise of transformation, or confront the challenges of conflict in his or her own role, it cannot be expected that the learning leader will be able to do so. This modeling of lived behavior is a critical coaching characteristic, especially in a time of great change. Since the language of change and transformation cannot always be clearly understood by others as they are moving through the change process, it is vital for the coach to be able to present a living example of confronting the vagaries of change and transformation. Not finding the appropriate words to describe or delineates change, feeling overwhelmed by the change events, being uncertain of the appropriate response are all normal role characteristics that can be used to school others, through modeling, how they can be addressed and incorporated into any change journey.

It is neither important nor appropriate for the coach to have all the answers. It is far more important to be delving into the right questions than it is to have the right answers to the wrong questions. The coach plays a dominant role in raising appropriate questions that relate to the experience of change and transformation as people accommodate new rules for work. As has been identified in other sections of this book, the work environment and all the elements related to the leader's understanding of context is becoming so different that the usual responses based on historical experiences are no longer acceptable for adequate problem solving. The coach, understanding this reality, creates a safe space for emerging concerns and challenges to be better addressed. Rather than eliminate the noise, anger, and aggravation of the transformation process, the coach uses those vagaries as tools, personal instruments that help people move through their own change experience. Exemplifying her or his own experience of challenge and of noise, the coach uses these experiences as vehicles for teaching and learning modeling for others, enabling others to engage new ways of doing business and undertaking the challenge of transforming clinical work.

In helping the learning leader accommodate his or her own struggle for change, the coach makes a safe space for that individual to address, give a voice to, and lay out the pain and struggle of adapting to change. The coach is receptive to the noise of learning as people confront the challenges of their own personal adaptations to change. The coach allows learning leaders both opportunity and time to express negative and painful experiences related to their own journey to effective leadership. The coach, by inviting this openness, creates a level of trust and interaction between coach and learner that makes a safe and productive learning experience for both.

ACTION LEARNING

The coach recognizes that learning best occurs in the process of action. Action learning reflects that the learning leader is an adult and will experience all that he or she needs in order to be able to undertake the appropriate role of leadership. The coach understands that the work environment creates all the opportunity necessary for learning leadership to unfold.

It is this notion, that the environment continually provides an opportunity for learning, that guides the coach in the role. As the change process unfolds and the environment begins to adjust, the conflict between past practices and future demand create the conditions within which new leadership is learned. Using these conditions, the coach develops scenarios and action processes that can be used in the learning dynamic to help the learning leader accommodate new rules and principles in the experience of applying new leadership processes in a changing world. It is this continuous and fluid change that creates the conditions within which contemporary leadership must unfold. The coach, using this fluid condition, challenges the learning leader to address the development of skills and talents within the context of a shifting reality. There is nothing less useful for the leader than a set of leadership skills in a context that cannot accommodate them. Furthermore, the learning leader must realize that leading others essentially involves unbundling others' attachment to their own work, providing a framework for new work, and bringing others into a new work environment able to practice their work with skill and competence. In addition, the learning leader must be able to help others in such a way that they can rise to the new work context and can to do their work with higher levels of satisfaction and with personal joy. There is nothing more challenging in the work of leadership than accomplishing these goals.

People will find changing to new practices difficult. This is normal and is to be expected in all phases of any work transformation. The challenge for the leader is to help others engage the demand for a changing practice by helping them visualize the need for that change and their own personal relationship to the change. They must begin to understand the series of steps that will be necessary for them to act on the demand for change. The time available for such activity is increasingly limited. As organizations compete and struggle to be successful in a new frame of reference for work, the timeline is shorter for accommodating the demand for change. That means that a part of the demand for work is the ability to adjust and change the capacity to work in "tighter" periods of time. The coach recognizes that she or he is not only helping others to change their relationship to work but also guiding them as to how to alter their way of confronting the change itself. The coach, in this set of circumstances reflects that *change itself is the work* and that commitment to the process of change is more important than commitment to any specific work function or activity. Since the work function or activity will change at any moment, the ability of the workers to adjust focus, attention, and effort quickly will be a critical part of their accommodation and adaptation to the change process. This expectation is appropriate for both coach and learning leader. Both must quickly adjust to their leadership practices as quickly as they expect workers to adjust their own work practices.

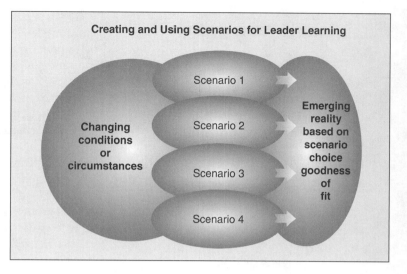

Creating and Using Scenarios for Leader Learning

Changing conditions or circumstances

Scenario 1
Scenario 2
Scenario 3
Scenario 4

Emerging reality based on scenario choice goodness of fit

Transitioning of Leader Skills

- Coach discusses various scenarios
- Dialogue centers on a vision of change
- Group process is facilitated
- Multiple insights are integrated
- Using a flipchart, perceptions are recorded
- Impact on leader role is outlined
- Skill deficits are defined
- Create work plan for matching skill with demand
- Compare learning work plan with each other
- Experiment and implement plan
- Evaluate in group progress and problems
- Revise and plan again, try again, review again

Change Itself is the Work

Both coaches and those they mentor must realize that in the time of great transformation the work of leadership is embedded in the change itself: recognizing change, acknowledging its impact on individuals and work, identifying and predicting the directions indicated by change, and remaining available to new insights and opportunities to literally see the change coming. Translating the elements of change into the action of work becomes the critical role of the leader, raising the level of accountability for matching performance to desired outcome in an ever-changing context for work.

Leader Discernment

Insightful
Future investment
Informed
Contemporary info.
Aware of surroundings
Intuitive
Sense context change
Integrates data
Sees inner "flow"

Leader Reflection

Can find a quiet place
Sorts through "noise"
Sees real from fad
Can link concepts
Touches internal values
Links broad notions
Trusts intuition
Sees the "river" of change
Finds direction
Gives change a language

Purposeful Questioning

The coach always assumes a questioning stance, recognizing that the right question is more important than the answer. Coaching questions are deliberate and focused:

- What is the direction of change?
- What are competencies of the learning leader?
- What is the fit between learner competencies and direction of change?
- What best exercise or learning opportunity fits the needs of the learner?
- Will learning tools will be required to facilitate the learning leader?
- What time and competency demands affect the rate of learning?
- What are the performance and outcome expectations for the learning leader?
- How will change in the learning leader be evaluated and sustained?

Leaders must be able to discern and reflect on the elements of change affecting leadership and work. The skill of reflection is a critical leadership talent often underaddressed. The wise leader recognizes the importance of being able to discern the correct fit between demand and response. As they increasingly emerge, there also is required a different response to that work. The coach with the learning leader must now take time to determine the relationship between demand and response.

The coach must be able to read the signposts of the change and to anticipate the implications of those changes on the role of leadership. The leader is always aware of the need to shift and adjust responses based on the change in expectations and performance. A part of this role in expressing leadership is found in the leader's facility with signpost reading and is grounded in the direction and pathway of change. The leader is able to understand the vectors for change and, in reading those vectors, can begin to determine the points of convergence that are indicated by the combined direction of each vector leading to an understanding of change. This signpost reading, or factoring, if you will, is an important leadership skill because it helps the leader anticipate the appropriateness and timing of responses. The coach requires in the learning leader an ability to read the signposts of change, to understand the compositions of movement that work in concert with each other, to be able to anticipate the appropriate responses driven by timing the events of change correctly and undertaking the appropriate action. This requires skill in reflection and discernment. The coach exemplifies this commitment through the use of dialogue and interaction. The dialogue and interaction and purposeful questioning and exploration become a subset of a directed conversation between coach and learning leader. The coach begins to work with the learning leader in a way that engages the issues as they are unfolding and invites to the table of discussion those players upon whom the change has the most impact or who have the most information related to the change. The wisdom that can be found through this collective dialogue and interaction by stakeholders begins to build an aggregate of appropriate responses. These new skills and opportunities create a database upon which the learning leader can draw as the issues demand and as the need arises. Developing skills and accessing and utilizing collective wisdom in decision making becomes a major strength and skill set of leaders as they mature and grow.

ACCOMMODATING INDIVIDUAL LEARNING NEEDS

The leader as coach recognizes that there are many ways of learning and of accommodating learning needs. All people are individuals. They have unique approaches to their own learning and development. What is critical for the coach is the commitment to the individual in addressing learning needs and committing to an ongoing program of learning. The coach enters this program of learning as a guide, helping individuals through their learning process with tools and techniques and an awareness that sometimes cannot be visualized within the learning moment. The coach recognizing the uniqueness of each individual learner, identifies with the learner a program of learning, reviews the processes related to the individual's best way of learning, and assesses situational and circumstantial tools and vehicles within which learning will unfold.

In the practice environment, the coach is predominantly a peer-based learner. The coach simply plays a role in helping others in their own commitment to learning and in their learning activities. The best model for this is the coach's own learning process and program. Through attending to his or her own leadership development, the coach exemplifies the elements, components, and processes associated with personal change and accommodation to transformation.

As a part of the coach's relationship with peers and learning leaders, dialogue is essential, since learning leadership and coaching involves the collective action of those members of the work team who continually relate to each other. It is appropriate that they understand their unique characteristics and practices and processes related to their own learning. This dialogue, facilitated by a good coach, helps people understand the activities and roles of others as they address their own learning processes. Furthermore, it gives all members of the team an opportunity to understand and accommodate the learning talents and unique skills of individual members.

As a part of this dynamic, the coach recognizes that each learning leader must have an action plan that relates specifically to his or her own pattern of learning and expectations for change. This coaching contract provides a framework for individual learner's to identify both their goals and their processes in a way that can be realistically yet rigorously applied.

A learning contract can either be a verbal or written agreement between coach and learning leader. If it is a group contract, it is an understanding between all the members of the learning group about their relationship to their learning goals and to facilitating each other's achievement of goals. Increasingly, coaching must involve more than a one-to-one relationship in a time of increasing pace and accelerating rate of change. The coach often cannot be spread thin enough to help guide others in their developmental work. As a result, a group work team contract with the coach is becoming a more common tool for transformational work.

The agreement is more a reflection of the relationship then it is of the coach's wisdom and expertise. In times of great change and personal transformation, every member of the team, including the coach, is fully on board with regard to personal change and transformation work. The coach essentially exemplifies the role of the chief learner, acting as the facilitator who calls to discussion all new learning that is necessary for learning leaders to move individually and in concert with each other.

Coaching in the new age calls for a commitment to help others transform. New rules and new roles in the 21st century call us to reconceptualize the function and role of leadership, as well as its impact on work organization and process. The leader is critical for organizations to successfully transform and attend to a completely different framework for work. The coach-learner relationship exemplifies a mutual commitment to the growth and development of new skills and talents in expressing leadership in this new age. It is an important vehicle for advancing the work of the organization, improving the dynamics of leadership, and providing a continuous opportunity for learning leadership to occur. This relationship is a positive vehicle for both coach and learner, ensuring competence in applying leadership in a time of great change when such leadership is desperately needed.

The Coach as Teacher

Coaching involves a program of learning, calling the coach to develop a systematic approach with the learner to guiding the learning leader on the developmental pathway. Critical elements of the program are:

- assessment of learning needs
- organized and systematic approach to learning
- a leadership learning plan
- identification of learning support systems
- formation of a learning contract
- clarification of the individual and group learning process
- timeline and program stages
- review and evaluation processes
- a definitive mechanism for ending the coaching relationship

---

Self-Directed Learning

The learner-coach arrangement is critical to the effectiveness of the learning process. This arrangement represents a partnership between two or more individuals who are committed to each other's learning, one being facilitator (coach) and the other being actor (learner). It is essential that they meet the basic requirements of a learning relationship in order to assure meaningful interaction and viable outcomes:

- the learner is always in control
- the coach is present for the learner's needs
- the learner is responsible for the outcomes of learning
- the processes of learning are always negotiated
- coaching is a learning partnership
- the coach is never a "parent"
- outcomes of learning are defined in advance
- an agreement of learning expectations is always explicit
- the learner determines when the coaching contract is ended
- the coach creates a safe milieu for honest dialogue
- learning evaluation is performance-based
- change is always the work of the learner

COACHING SCENARIO 1: TEAM-BASED ISSUES

Jill was struggling to keep up with the demands of the team. The learning team had been organized as a way of building mentor support for new charge nurses who were emerging into very new leadership roles. Most of the charge nurses on the team had not been in the role for

continues

Coaching-Group Learning Contract

Components:

- mutual goals are defined
- collective agreement regarding outcomes
- regularly scheduled group process times
- continuous peer evaluation
- peers control group membership
- members contract performance expectations
- defining the timeline for performance

Relationship

- agreement to support each other
- evaluations are developmental
- regular group process
- dialogue leads to change
- trusting and interdependent

Outcomes

- individuals feel valued
- performance has improved
- personal and team expectations are met
- developmental learning is shared
- learners themselves become coaches

COACHING SENARIO 1: TEAM-BASED ISSUES *continued*

more than a year and had been in practice for less than five years. Each member of the team had committed to partnering with others in identifying leadership needs and skills necessary to be effective in the leadership role. The group gathered together with their coach bimonthly to deal with specific leadership development issues and to evaluate progress.

Team members had made progress, but Jill felt herself falling behind. It seemed that other team members were growing at a faster rate and catching on to the leadership role more quickly than Jill was. Whenever Jill brought up issues it seemed as though they held the team back from consideration of more important or advanced concerns. The last time the learning team had gathered together, Jill had felt a real sense of their irritation with her and the questions she raised. The coach had pulled Jill aside following the meeting and asked Jill how she felt she was progressing and if she desired additional personal time with the coach. Jill was uncertain as to whether that meant the coach felt she was lagging behind and needed special individual attention. She certainly did not want to hold the team back. Indeed, Jill was concerned whether she fit the role she was attempting to undertake and whether she should simply withdraw from the team and, ultimately, from the role.

Scenario evaluation

In the group, discuss Jill's circumstances. Identify the issues that Jill expresses and make some assumptions about the underlying issues that your team identifies may be affecting Jill's progress. In addition, explore Jill's circumstances by answering the following questions:

1. How did Jill fall behind without other members of the team recognizing it?
2. What was the learning team's obligation as Jill fell behind?
3. Was there something the learning team could have done to be of more assistance to Jill?
4. What is the coach's role with regard to both Jill and the learning team?
5. Can Jill be rescued from these circumstances, or should she move out of the role?

Break into small teams and devise a team contract and a specific learning plan for Jill that follows up on this set of circumstances. Be creative and enumerate what you feel is the coach's role and how that role can facilitate Jill's progress. Report back to the whole group and collectively agree upon the next step for both the coach and for Jill.

COACHING SCENARIO 2: ESTABLISHING THE COACHING RELATIONSHIP

Ben has just been promoted to his first management position. Ben is a little concerned about how the management position and his skills will match. Never having been a manager before, Ben feels a tremendous need for growth and development in the role. Yet, he has to land on the ground running since he is already in the role, not leaving much time for learning.

continues

COACHING SENARIO 2: ESTABLISHING THE COACHING RELATIONSHIP *continued*

Ben has a great deal of respect for his previous manager, Sandra. One day over coffee, Ben and Sandra discussed Ben's new role as manager. During the conversation Ben asked Sandra if she would mind acting as a coach and mentor for him as he began the role of manager. Ben pointed out to Sandra that, while the basics certainly were in place, there were problems and issues that may arise from time to time for which he would need advice and counsel. Neither Ben nor Sandra had been in a coaching and mentoring relationship before. Sandra was a little concerned as to whether she would be competent in providing insight and guidance to Ben. She was also a little concerned as to how the relationship should be established and what the characteristics should be that defined the coaching relationship. Sandra left her lunch with Ben wondering what her first steps should be.

Scenario exploration

As a learning team, gather together to discuss and expand on Ben's situation. Spend some time conversing about Sandra's position and the contribution that she might be able to make to Ben. Respond to the following questions:

1. What should Ben ask and/or expect from Sandra?
2. What are the basic elements of the coaching/mentoring relationship?
3. Should the coaching relationship be narrowly defined, or should it be open, available to all issues and circumstances?
4. Explain the pros and cons of a written versus verbal coaching relationship.
5. In Ben and Sandra's circumstances, what are the clear outcomes that can be defined as a result of their coaching relationship?

Break up into small groups and prepare a coaching contract for Ben and Sandra. When you have prepared it for them, compare the contract elements you have constructed, evaluate them, and together create a learning agreement for Ben and Sandra with which you can all agree.

Elements of the Coaching Agreement

The coaching contract needs to contain specific elements in order for it to adequately address the individual performance roles and expectations of the parties to the coaching experience.

1. The coaching contract should define the role expectations of both coach and leadership learner. The role expectations and the obligations of commitments made to each other are a critical part of the faithfulness each has to the growth of leadership and the skill development both in coaching and in leader development. This contract, which enumerates the expectations of each to the other, helps provide a framework within which both can perform and meet the commitments of their coaching relationship.

2. The coaching contract should enumerate the expectations for performance and for outcome. The agreement between coach and learning leader is one that is directed toward achieving some specific value for performance outcome. This expectation should be clearly enough enumerated so that it can be identified as a part of the expectation that each has for the other. Failing to accomplish the goals of coaching and learning leadership does not reflect well on the coaching/mentoring experience. In fact, it may indicate that no real coaching relationship existed. Identifying a specific performance expectation and its relationship to mutually desired or defined outcomes helps discipline the relationship and maintain its meaning and impact as it unfolds.

3. Any coaching contract should have some elements of measurement of performance and accomplishment of goals. Here again, the coach/mentor relationship cannot have much value or impact if some differences are maintained through the process of coaching and learning development. Points of demarcation, elements of evaluation, review of degrees of improvement or change over time all help the learner meet performance expectations and advances the relationship between coach and learning leader. Such evaluation keeps the process focused and directed toward specific goals and performance expectations and assures that the relationship remains one that is developmental, productive, and growth oriented.

4. A timeframe should be created for the expectations of performance so that accomplishment or changes in practices or behaviors can be defined within a specific timeframe. This helps discipline the expectations for performance and begins to set parameters around

actual change behavior. Often in the coaching and learning relationship there is an open timeframe with regard to performance expectations and specific changes. The problem with this is that specific changes may not ever occur as a product of the relationship. What results instead is a high level of personal relationship interaction and a low level of substantive change and role impact. Developing friendships and an abiding relationship between coach and learning leader may be a valuable human experience, but does not necessarily advance the development of effective leadership skills or roles.

5. The coach-learner role should at some time come to an end with regard to its formal purpose and mentoring interaction. This is not to suggest that the relationship between people ever end. However, what is important is to recognize that the coach and learner role is purposeful and directed toward achieving meaningful and viable products. It is when these ends are obtained and development has occurred and expected changes happen, as enumerated in the role contract, that the relationship changes its form as well as its purpose. Reflecting this understanding of the change in form and purpose, the contract enumerates a time when its formal nature ends and the expectations for the agreement have been fulfilled. This gives both coach and learner an opportunity to evaluate the effectiveness of their interaction, to determine the value of its impact on expectations, and to evaluate the outcomes and impact of the coaching relationship. In this way the real value of the coaching relationship is clearly spelled out and identified with the specific outcomes involved as a result of the contracted interaction.

SUGGESTED READINGS

1. Anderson, M. C. (2003). *Bottom-line organization development: Implementing and evaluating strategic change for lasting value.* Boston: Butterworth-Heinemann.
2. Bacon, T. R., & Spear, K. I. (2003). *Adaptive coaching: The art and practice of a client-centered approach to performance improvement.* Palo Alto, CA: Davies-Black.
3. Bench, M. (2003). *Career coaching: An insider's guide.* Palo Alto, CA: Davies-Black.
4. Carter, L., Giber, D. J., & Goldsmith, M. (2001). *Best practices in organization development and change: Culture, leadership, retention, performance, coaching; case studies, tools, models, research.* San Francisco: Jossey-Bass.
5. Cloke, K., & Goldsmith, J. (2003). *The art of waking people up: Cultivating awareness and authenticity at work.* San Francisco: Jossey-Bass.
6. Coens, T., & Jenkins, M. (2000). *Abolishing performance appraisals: Why they backfire and what to do instead.* San Francisco: Berrett-Koehler Publishers.
7. Cullen, J., & D'Innocenzo, L. (1999). *The agile manager's guide to coaching to maximize performance.* Bristol, VT: Velocity Business Publishers.
8. Dotlich, D. L., & Cairo, P. C. (1999). *Action coaching: How to leverage individual performance for company success.* San Francisco: Jossey-Bass.
9. Flaherty, J. (1999). *Coaching: Evoking excellence in others.* Boston: Butterworth-Heinemann.
10. Fournies, F. F. (2000). *Coaching for improved work performance* (Rev. ed.). New York: McGraw-Hill.
11. Goldsmith, M., Lyons, L., & Freas, A. (2000). *Coaching for leadership: How the world's greatest coaches help leaders learn.* San Francisco: Jossey Bass/Pfeiffer.
12. Kamp, D. (1999). *The 21st-century manager: Future-focused skills for the next millennium.* Dover, NH: Kogan Page.
13. Lenhardt, V. (2004). *Coaching for meaning: The culture and practice of coaching and team building.* New York: Palgrave Macmillan.
14. Markle, G. L. (2000). *Catalytic coaching: The end of the performance review.* Westport, CT: Quorum Books.
15. Parsloe, E., & Wray, M. J. (2000). *Coaching and mentoring: Practical methods to improve learning.* Sterling, VA: Kogan Page.
16. Stone, F. M. (1999). *Coaching, counseling & mentoring: How to choose & use the right technique to boost employee performance.* New York: Amacom.
17. Stone, F. M. (2002). *Coaching and mentoring.* Oxford: Capstone.

18. Thorpe, S., & Clifford, J. (2003). *The coaching handbook: An action kit for trainers & managers*. Sterling, VA: Kogan Page.

19. Warner, J. (2002). *Aspirations of greatness: Mapping the midlife leader's reconnection to self and soul*. New York: John Wiley.

20. Weiss, T. B., & Kolberg, S. (2003). *Coaching competencies and corporate leadership*. Boca Raton, FL: St. Lucie Press.

21. Whitmore, J. (2002). *Coaching for performance: Growing people, performance and purpose* (3rd ed.). Naperville, IL: Nicholas Brealey.

CHAPTER 9

Leading with Courage

CHAPTER OBJECTIVES:

Upon completion of this chapter, the reader will:

1. Discuss the significance of revolutionary behaviors as a vehicle to continuing adaptation and transition into the information age.
2. Understand the value of courageous leader behaviors and their impact on organizational performance.
3. Enumerate four strategies to develop courageous communication competence.
4. Identify specific leader behaviors that reflect courage.

INTRODUCTION

The paradox of leadership requires leaders to be creative and futuristic in their thinking while sustaining the essence of the current culture, which may be fixed and entrenched. This challenge finds leaders often stuck, sustaining the past at the expense of adapting to the changing external environment. Leading courageously requires specific skills and focus on work, in which the leader neither dwells in the past nor revels in the present. The courageous leader fully understands personal strengths and weaknesses and how best to use those skills in addressing the obstacles to the future, and moves forward assertively to cocreate the preferred future that reflects emerging expectations, new knowledge, and new technology.

In this chapter, leaders will examine the nature of courage from several perspectives. A description of the courageous leader as a revolutionary is presented from Kuhn's (1996) perspective of scientific revolutions and the phenomena surrounding the emergence of new science and new models. Several communication challenges that continually confront leaders and require much courage are presented to further examine the essence of courage and stimulate discussion. In the final section, specific challenges reflecting leader courage are offered to leaders to continue their courageous journey of health-care leadership.

> **Quantum Gem**
>
> The most radical revolutionary will become a conservative the day after the revolution.
>
> Hannah Arendt

Facing Fear

I have not ceased being fearful, but I have ceased to let fear control me. I have accepted fear as a part of life—specifically the fear of change, the fear of the unknown; and I have gone ahead despite the pounding in my heart that says: turn back, turn back, you'll die if you venture too far.

Erica Jong

Courage

I do not ask to walk smooth paths, nor bear an easy load

I pray for strength and fortitude to climb the rock strewn road.

Give me such courage and I can scale the hardest peaks alone,

And transform every stumbling block into a stepping stone!

Gail Brook Burket

Courage

Few people realize that Ford Motor Company was Henry Ford's third attempt at making automobiles. He was voted out in one company and went bankrupt in another. He was ousted from the Henry Ford Company when he insisted on improving the design of the car instead of thinking of short-term profits. When he was removed by the board of directors, the name was changed to the Cadillac Automotive Company. The Cadillac was originally a Ford. Later, as we all know, Ford's quest for a better car paid off.

Dare to Revolutionize

The work expected of the leader is analogous to the scientific revolution described by Kuhn (1996) in the *Structure of Scientific Revolutions*. As the world evolves from the industrial age to the information age, the work of health care is shifting from work that requires the skill set of an employee to work that requires the skill set of the knowledge worker. Previously, the work of the employee was grounded in functional analysis, manual dexterity, fixed skill sets, an emphasis of process value and practice, and unilateral performance. This is quite different from the required skills of the knowledge worker, namely, the ability to synthesize concepts, embody multiple intelligences, demonstrate competence in providing care, skill set mobility, being driven by outcomes that create value, and the ability to function most effectively within a team model.

While the evolution to the knowledge worker paradigm may seem slow, even invisible, there is a revolution of work processes occurring. This revolution occurs through courageous leaders committed to the belief that the creation of anomalous situations, or situations that deviate from the norm, is essential to facilitate the paradigm shift from the industrial age to the information age.

Quantum leaders thrive in the work of discovery, which includes asking new questions, identifying new methods to examine processes, finding new areas of relevance, and creating new meaning for the work of health care. These processes necessarily challenge the current assumptions and industrial paradigm underpinning health care, creating the well-known *anomaly* or shift in scientific knowledge that changes shared assumptions and subverts existing traditions of practice. In time, the anomaly created by courageous health-care leaders will evolve into a scientific revolution and traditions will be shattered, thus rendering the tradition-bound activity of the current paradigm inappropriate. It is important to note that the courageous leader who assumes the role of the *anomaly creator* can be often lonely and sometimes scorned. However, it is only through the creation of an anomaly that new realities can be advanced and ultimately supported. New ideas tend to emerge only with difficulty in cultures strongly entrenched in current processes. Resistance is the norm to most new ideas.

Creating a sustainable revolution will result in certain outcomes. First, the current paradigm must be replaced in whole or part by an incompatible new one; second, the new approach is immune to attack by competent knowledge owners. The journey of the courageous leader is never finished. As the courageous leader moves forward and continually examines personal behaviors, values, and communication processes, new paradigms result in better ways to conceptualize and provide health care.

In summary, several challenges always remain with the leader committed to the revolution of health care. These include:

- Creation of a new reality that is better than the current reality in some way
- Appreciation for current dogma, and willingness and courage to remove existing assumptions
- Commitment to changing the culture or social behaviors necessary for revolutions to succeed
- Tolerance of rejection
- Appreciation of areas of vulnerability
- Avoidance of acquiescing to the glamour of short-lived fads instead of a substantive, sustainable revolution
- Willingness to abandon the past
- Developing energy to sustain emerging revolutionary outcomes and continually move forward

An example of a paradigm shift can be found in the changing documentation of health-care records. Computerized word processing has all but eliminated the need for the typewriter and caregiver handwriting. The paradigm shift began with upgrade from a manual typewriter to an electric typewriter, which enhanced the processes within the current paradigm of creating legible documents. The work of documentation has been transformed from a single, static entry of information to an electronic entry that is retrievable, editable, and stored as long as the author wishes and not simply modified from a handwritten entry to a typewriter entry.

The shift from invasive surgery to the use of external scope-facilitated procedures is another example of the beginning of a paradigm shift: less invasive procedures, different equipment needed, differing skills needed to complete the processes. The role of the physician and nurse has changed dramatically in this transformation, one that is incomplete, as the need for some invasive procedures still exists. The work of invasive surgery has yet to be completely replaced. As imaging technology continues to advance, the anomaly of the noninvasive procedure will become the dominant paradigm once biological and genomic therapies further complete the transformation to surgical interventions that are exclusively noninvasive.

Build a Conspiracy of Innovation

As previously noted, the journey of transformation is often paradoxical; people actively support the idea of and need for new processes and strategies, but seldom dedicate adequate time or energy to live the role of transformer. Excessively high workloads take precedence over reflective time for examination of work effectiveness and evaluation of opportunities for change. Nurses have demonstrated the ability to adapt to differing circumstances but have not demonstrated this ability as a discipline to embrace and engage in change processes. Most likely, this is due to the lack of skills in translating great clinical ideas into ways of doing business in an economically driven marketplace. The need emerges for courageous leaders to build conspiracies for innovation, to gather a critical group of people committed to seeing the good ideas through to actualization, to create passion for the work that will overcome the obstacles, and to develop relationship skills that will place the right people in the right place at the right time (Porter-O'Grady, 2003). Courageous leaders committed to innovation demonstrate the ability to manage the noise created by anomalous processes, develop a few key players, and plan or conspire to work through others to advance the innovation throughout the system. The effective leader recognizes that innovative ideas are seldom spontaneous; rather, they occur through methodical processes of creating evidence for the idea and cascading support from those in the organization. This is an often slow and lonely process. In the next section, several behaviors are presented to assist leaders dedicated to the transformation of practice through innovation.

The Daring Leader

Often times, the creative and innovative leader is described as outrageous or gutsy. According to Frieberg & Frieberg (2004), gutsy leaders are not afraid of criticism or ridicule by others. They have dismantled fear-based behaviors and processes and replaced them with heart, soul, discipline, loyalty, humor, and of course, long-term record profits. While it might seem contradictory to have gutsy leaders in health care, where the stakes of life and health are significant and the need for consistently high-quality outcomes are expected, the reality is that current processes

---

Courage to Risk

To laugh is to risk appearing the fool.

To weep is to risk appearing sentimental.

To reach for another is to risk involvement.

To expose your feelings is to risk exposing your true self.

To place your ideas, your dreams before a crowd is to risk their loss.

To love is to risk not being loved in return.

To live is to risk dying.

To believe is to risk despair.

To try is to risk failure.

But risks must be taken, because the greatest hazard in life is to risk nothing.

The person who risks nothing, does nothing, has nothing, is nothing. They may avoid suffering and sorrow, but they cannot learn, feel change, grow, love, live.

Chained by their attitudes they are slaves; they have forfeited their freedom.

Only a person who risks is free.

Anonymous Chicago Teacher

Gem

The art of progress is to preserve order amid change and to preserve change amid order.

Alfred North Whitehead

have yet to achieve the desired outcomes. Significant modifications of the health-care system are still desperately needed to both create the desired outcomes and to effectively transform the system into the new age of technology and meet the greater expectations for high-quality, caring, therapeutic relationships. Consumers are demanding compassionate health care with the best of technology at a reasonable price; thus the need for much more innovation and transformation of current practices. Gusty leaders have several things in common (Frieberg & Frieberg, 2004). These include:

- An emphasis to ensure that employees are overwhelmingly enthusiastic about their organization, not just satisfied
- Promoting of a sense of ownership of the work; those closest to the point of care are recognized as the experts of the organization
- Building business literacy competency among all employees; developing skills in translating individual work through accounting processes to the bottom line of the organization and the employee paycheck
- Expecting accountability for success and failures through service guarantees
- Creating a moral imperative for doing great work for the right reason: work is more than just a job
- The ability to stand up for what is right and to admit mistakes in front of those you work with and to say *I don't know when you don't!*

The Vigilant Leader

In addition to being gusty, the courageous leader must also be vigilant of the context in which care is provided and the interrelated components in the environment. Clinical vigilance is recognized as a key behavior in minimizing failures to rescue and thus improve patient outcomes. When a nurse is vigilant, he or she is likely to intervene on the patient's behalf, recognize problems early, or avert them entirely. Emerick (2004) writes, "vigilance is a collection of behaviors and activities, based on professional commitment or duty, that includes seeking or intellectually scanning within the nurse-patient relationship for situations that require nursing actions and reacting appropriately to that need." Vigilance is one of the caring acts of nursing that are deeply ingrained into the professional role and are often undetected by non-nurses. These acts often seem intangible and nonspecific, are identified as lower priority in skill development, and marginalize nursing's artful practice to the demands of efficiency and cost control.

Historically, the notions of vigilance emanate from the work of Fairman (1992) and the rationale for the creation of intensive care units. Specialized knowledge was needed, as was more frequent monitoring, identification of high-risk situations, and timely actions. Kennedy (2000) further described vigilance as a means to support normalcy, rather than a search for pathology, requiring confidence, intelligence, intellectual curiosity, and objectivity to assess the situation. Another significant attribute of vigilance is the act of *doing nothing well*: allowing events to progress naturally when the range of normalcy is identified. Knowing when to intervene and not to intervene is critical for the courageous leader; it involves leader actions of trusting, being competent, and recognizing past experiences of the team.

Similarly, there are opportunities for leader vigilance in ensuring that the infrastructure to support clinical vigilance is in place and is able to support current safe practice and innovation. Leader vigilance is about the commitment to leadership through the specialized knowledge of the organization's infrastructure, processes and outcomes, routine assessment of processes and outcomes, recognition of high-risk situations, and timely reaction to avoid negative outcomes. Leader vigilance, as expression of courageous leader behaviors, is more than sensitivity for conditions that will lead to error; it means being proactive rather than reactive in assuring that the conditions for innovation and quality work are always present. Leader vigilance means scanning for opportunities and taking action to advance both the work of the organization and the practice of nursing. Leader vigilance is truly an art form of nursing leadership that embodies a high level of awareness for the signals that indicate effectiveness and excellence. Those signals reflect minor variations that could lead to major issues if not investigated, and the leader must have the courage to react at the appropriate time. The characteristics and representative behaviors of leader vigilance include the following:

- Discusses minor issues regularly with employees
- Recognizes potential problems early
- Intervenes on the employees behalf
- Builds sustainable relationship with employees
- Early elimination of outdated practices
- Early adoption of contemporary practices more suited to the context of health care

Diminished vigilance is described as incomplete vigilance relative to one of the basic components of vigilance, such as intellectually scanning the work of nursing, identifying areas for intervention or nonintervention, and reacting appropriately. An action reflecting diminished vigilance may be the result of poor judgment due to inappropriate or lack of knowledge, failure to scan the environment appropriately, or failure to react in a timely manner. Examples of diminished vigilance include:

- Inappropriate actions taken due to lack of knowledge
- Interventions that focus only on the immediate issues and do not address the situation effectively
- Undermonitoring of the critical elements of practice
- Inappropriate judgment as to the appropriate intervention to be taken or not taken
- Failure to prevent negative outcomes

Non-vigilance is the absence of professional commitment that precludes the nurse from being vigilant, namely intellectually able to scan for the critical indicators of work effectiveness and to react appropriately. Examples of the outcomes of non-vigilance include:

- Negative patient outcomes
- Negative employee outcomes
- Poor leader-employee relationships
- Potential problems become real problems
- Failure to recognize problem behaviors
- Failure to respond to significant data, leading to errors and missed signs and symptoms
- Lack of awareness of appropriate delegation practices specific to clinical and managerial tasks
- Lack of awareness of the impact of the level of secretarial support

One of the challenges for leadership is how to integrate the essence of clinical vigilance into productivity systems, or, how does one make the business case for vigilance? Historically, productivity measurement has

---

Leader Vigilance Data Scanning

- Status of available staff at the aggregate and daily level
- Status of supply availability
- Working relationships between departments
- Presence of joy in the patient care area
- Presence of joy in the break room
- Patient satisfaction and perception of patient care; perception of the health-care experience
- Productivity measures that include variance analysis from volume and projected costs
- Occurrence reports
- Skill level of available staff
- Errors/failure to rescue situations
- Informal staff feedback—ask focused questions rather than general satisfaction questions

not included calculation of preventive measures, a significant component of the nursing role. This is not because clinical vigilance has been ignored or disregarded; rather, it is because those accountable for vigilance have not been able to create objective and defensible measures that can be integrated into a productivity system. Recent published research documents the impact of registered nurse oversight and monitoring and the resultant *rescuing* of patients from negative consequences. According to Blakeney (2003), ANA president, the challenge is not reinventing how nursing is practiced, but how nursing is perceived and partnered within health-care institutions. The perception of rescuing, observing the subtle changes, and continuous vigilance needs to be translated into current productivity measurement systems. While good nursing care is often seen through the absence of problems, this "essence" requires credible, standard metrics not currently available in most productivity monitoring systems. Measuring success on the basis of events that do not occur is possible, given the recent publications specific to pressure ulcers, nosocomial pneumonia, patient falls, and urinary tract infections. Thus the new metrics that identify the time and skill level for the definition and articulation of the minimum monitoring necessary for safe patient outcomes must be created and become an essential element in the calculations of caregiver productivity.

Dare to Revive the Nursing Uniform

Letting go of the past requires careful analysis of what we are giving up and what should be retained, which is a process of using resources more appropriately and finding better value for one's efforts. A revolution in nurse uniforms is in the making. New technology and new environmental hazards have rendered the current nurse uniform only marginally helpful to the work of nursing.

Uniforms are immediate identifiers. They represent authority and convey a sense of competency within the nursing field. The once-traditional white uniform, white stockings, and starched cap of nurses has been unceremoniously replaced with bright and colorful uniforms. Both licensed and nonlicensed caregivers have adopted similar uniforms, diminishing the use of the uniform as an identifier of the nurse.

In the spirit of creativity and utility, members of the Fabric Workshops and Museum (FWM), in association with the Center for the Study of the History of Nursing, have examined nurse uniforms and proposed a future uniform that combines the lore of science fiction with new material technologies (Houweling, 2004). Conductive fiber technologies embedded in the fabric equip it to assess a patient's vital signs at the touch of a hand. It also provides hazard protection from a biological attack or biological spill, which enables nurses to administer to patients without endangering themselves.

A computer-generated model of the "Intergalactic Nurse" uses a uniform design incorporating the acupuncture concept of *chi* (energy flow) (Houweling, 2004). The uniform conceptualized for nursing in the 23rd century incorporates reflective tape, magnets, and silver-plated fiber that can be wired for computers or other electronics. The antimicrobial fabric conducts heat via silver to soothe the body at the various chi points, further supporting the safe practice of nursing. The design, a collaborative effort of artists Puett, Dion, and Kerr, the Fabric Workshop and Museum in Philadelphia, and materials from 3M, Sauquoit Industries, and Noble Fiber Technologies, is an example of creativity, evidence-based decision making, and courage to change the present paradigm on the basis of the new nursing role expectations and the new hazards of the work.

Quantum Gem

Over the last 20 years, we've changed the world just enough to make it radically different, but not enough to make it work.

Anna Quindlen

Discussion

Consider the changing role of the nurse leader.

How would you design the "uniform" or the basic competencies of the leader to reflect the needs of the 23rd century in a technologically healing context?

What knowledge would be essential for the processes of rework?

What protective skills would be necessary for the leader?

What would you leave behind that would not compromise the future value of nursing?

Revolutionizing the uniform for the nurse may indeed be much less complicated than reworking the cultural context of the work of nursing. The courageous leader approaches rework in spite of its awesome and overwhelming nature; the courageous leader moves forward because it is the right thing to do.

COURAGEOUS COMMUNICATION

Courageous leaders continually work to communicate openly and honestly, even in the most unpleasant situations. The skills of confronting, sharing information, ending relationships, and using new technology effectively are presented in this section as guides for continuing the evolving journey to excellence.

Dare to Confront

It is trite to say that delivering unpleasant news is seldom easy, given that so many leaders continue to struggle with sharing honest, open, and caring communication. Numerous explanations for less-than-open communication have been identified and include lack of skill in confronting difficult issues, reluctance to upset the other person, unwillingness to stand out in a group, and fear of retaliation. Many strategies to confront others as caring actions have been recommended, such as skill-building workshops and increasing individual accountability as a core performance expectation. Yet, the challenge remains. There may be no other skill that requires as much courage as giving unpleasant, but honest, feedback.

Courageous leaders have no magic strategies; rather, they practice, practice, and practice some more in giving feedback to others in the most timely and caring manner.

Consider the situation in which a recently hired surgical director has been noted to be confrontational and has not been listening to others during introductory meetings. The supervisor shares the feedback and after discussion with the director advises her that this behavior is inconsistent with the culture of the organization and needs to be modified. Within two days, more feedback is received of the same negative nature. The supervisor does not wait for change to occur but rather once again informs the director of the poor communication style. Both expectations for change and strategies to support better communication are discussed. The first confrontation was a challenge, but the second was even more difficult. Failing to follow through on issues as they recur results in unresolved, festering issues that eventually result in a critical incident. Courageous leaders focus on addressing issues quickly and appropriately as a key strategy to role model expectations and to support open dialogue and effective teamwork.

Dare to Tell All

As more and more health-care information is available and managed through the Internet, leaders are presented a new challenge of ensuring that the right information is shared with the right person at the right time. Legislation to limit the sharing of patient information and expectations from employees to know what is going on often seem contradictory. The principles of information-sharing specific to patient information has been defined in recent HIPPA legislation; only the patient or those designated by the patient have access to the information and are able to discuss patient information.

> ### Gem
> Success is measured not so much by the position that one has reached in life as by the obstacles which he has overcome while trying to succeed.
>
> Booker T. Washington

> ### Quantum Gem
> There is a fine line between healthy dissent and arrogant disregard for authority.
>
> Pamela Herr

> ### Gem
> It is better to be a lion for a day than to be a sheep all your life.
>
> Sister Elizabeth Kenny

Discussion

Dare to Tell ALL

Much information about department or organizational operations is believed confidential. As a leader you are entrusted with information specific to clinical management, policies, pay structures, discipline criteria, costs of care, supplies, and equipment, to name a few. Carefully review the information and determine how much of the information you can share with every member of your department. When you identify information that is not currently shared but you believe should be, use your newly acquired skills in being a courageous leader and work to change the expectation to allow information sharing.

Who will support your recommendation?

What are the barriers that must be overcome?

Quantum Gem

Changes are not only possible and predictable, but to deny them is to be an accomplice to one's own unnecessary vegetation.

Gail Sheehy

Knowing which information specific to organizational operations that can be shared with employees continues to challenge leaders. Telling all is irresponsible, and sharing nothing is paralyzing. Guidelines are needed that maximize employee involvement, protect employee confidentiality, and addresses the evolving nature of data. Hesselbein (2004) has noted that rigid hierarchies, which assign people boxes and restrict information to assigned boxes, up-down, superior-subordinate relationships, are disappearing from the world of effective organizations. The new reality of fluid, flexible management systems, structures, and practices requires an inclusive, circular organizational culture in which information is shared openly with those involved in the work of the organization. The inclusionary approach reinforces that an inclusionary culture is indeed about the beliefs and values practiced by all members of the organization, not just a selected few in selected boxes.

New energy and synergy emerge when organizations share operational information specific to revenues, expenses, outcomes, and strategies. In essence, leadership becomes dispersed throughout the organization, and involvement and support for the organization increases exponentially with the circle of inclusion approach. This is much different from the old departmental or boxes of control that expected communication separation and isolation. Managing from a circular model moves the organization to new levels of engagement, inquiry, performance, and results.

Dare to Move to Virtual Communication

The increasing use of electronic communication creates opportunities for increased collaboration, participation of all team members, and significant decreases of travel time to and from meetings. Online education programs have pioneered the model which results in an increased level of student participation with the required posting of ideas and feedback to reflect assimilation and comprehension of assigned materials. These processes are readily applicable to organizational group communication in which input from each participant is needed. Courageous leaders have challenged the traditional face-to-face meetings and developed new meeting processes with clear guidelines to assure the desired outcomes are achieved. Examples of guidelines to transform meeting processes to a more effective and efficient use of time and energy include:

- All meetings will be virtual unless there is specific, identified benefit to physical presence; first and last meetings are in person to establish relationships and celebrate completion
- Identification of required participants
- Clear expectations for each member to participate and provide feedback/discussion for all issues in virtual work
- Specific time frames for project discussion and completion
- Completion of a standard evaluation for each virtual meeting

Dare to Close with Closure

Most leaders have experienced relationships that did not end well. Miscommunications, differing values, competing interests, or decision-making styles were just too different to reside together. Chinn (2004) tells us that ending relationships or asking a member to leave a group can be appropriate. As difficult as that might be, sometimes the work of the group and the individual are not harmonious. When attempts to address the differences are not successful, actions must be taken to sustain overall group effectiveness. It is unrealistic to think that everyone can live together happily ever after; this is just not consistent with reality. This is not to say the relationship was a failure; rather, one phase is ending and another is beginning. Courage is certainly required to address the issue and move on as kindly as possible. Allowing the conflict or disharmony to fester and failing to address it is less than courageous and may in fact border on cowardice!

COURAGEOUS LEADER BEHAVIORS

Dare to Rework the Work

The context for all health-care service must change and adapt as rapidly as new technologies, pharmaceuticals, and genome innovations, which are forever changing the delivery of care. Courageous leaders are focused on advancing the practice setting to accommodate new processes and achieving the work of the day. Assumptions are challenged and rationales are validated to ensure that changes are appropriate and ahead of the curve. The courageous leader seldom waits for others to lead the way with new innovations and completion of process validation. Being a part of designing the future is an essential role for both the leader and members of the organization.

> **Gem**
>
> Life is a grindstone. Whether it grinds you down or polishes you up depends on what you are made of.
>
> Anonymous

Dare to Eliminate Your Job

As the nature of work changes, few current jobs should remain as they are. For example, using oral thermometers, sippy diets for ulcer management, and invasive chest surgeries have been replaced by ear thermometers, pharmaceuticals to control gastric acid, and endoscopic procedures that are safer and more efficient. The same evolution, while not as dramatic, is occurring for leaders. Classroom orientation has been replaced by online courses, communication has moved from phones to e-mail, and manual calculators have been replaced by complex software calculation programs. Eliminating the specific tasks but not the basic work is the challenge faced by all leaders: the work of nursing assessment, planning, intervention, and evaluation remains, while the time and tools to complete the processes evolve continually. The need for employee performance reviews is a constant, but the content, method, and frequency of the process evolves as well. No employee should have the same type of evaluation as occurred 10 years ago. Reworking the job description on a regular basis to reflect the desired outcomes of the work, not the specific approach, is an evolving process. As with the virtual meeting processes, leaders continue to ensure effective communication but move from processes that may overuse resources and decrease the number of participants, and towards better processes that result in better discussion and outcomes. For example, if the majority of new employee orientation can be online, the space requirement for classrooms decreases significantly but the need for computer terminals increases. The expectation for a quality orientation that produces competent caregivers never varies; the methods and tools used to achieve the competence often change based on advances. The leader must continually evaluate all processes and eliminate the outdated jobs while sustaining the essential values of quality, integrity, and efficiency of resource use.

Caution is noted regarding frequent changes in organizational reporting structures as the means to advance practice. Rearranging processes is much different from evolving and transforming processes. Too often, new organizational structures are created to manage unsatisfactory performance of certain individuals. Courageous leaders learn to confront the issues and avoid making complex system changes that serve only to confuse others in the organization. Only when leaders truly believe that the future is advanced should changes be made in the organizational chart.

As leaders rework the work, the significance and number of policies should be examined as well. Too often, policies that are long out of date are retained in the system for no apparent reason. All leaders should be challenged to eliminate or archive at least two policies for each new one created.

Dare to Live in the World of Information Technology

The complexities of information technology have caused much confusion for nurse leaders, who must integrate computerized systems into the work of nursing. While much has been gained in the cross-training of nursing and information technology skills, significant work remain to transform today's nurses to tech-savvy clinicians. Given that computerization is here to stay and there is no turning back to a manual world, and given the pervasiveness of computerization, the courageous leader must recognize the need to immerse him- or herself into the discipline of information technology and become tech-savvy. A toolbox of resources that guide leaders in understanding basic computer function, networking, web-based learning, Internet programs, and technical support to assure adequate functioning of computerized systems are essential skills for the quantum leader. This is not to say that leaders should develop skills in programming. They should develop expertise in the management of existing systems and the evaluation of new technology that will serve to enhance practice, rather than merely accept an additional level of computerization without specific clinical benefits.

Dare to Transform the Culture

Seldom does a leader have the opportunity to start with a new facility and create a new culture for the provision of health-care services. However, whenever the opportunity is present for a new facility or for a new unit, it is courageous to embrace a process of CARE transformation that redesigns processes to address the problems and inefficiencies of the current system. More often than not, new construction and renovations focus on duplicating the current physical environment with only minor modifications of existing care processes. The opportunities are incredible for creating a better future that requires caregivers to examine their practice, recommit to doing the right thing for the right reason, and to improve personal satisfaction with the organization, which must translate to quality patient outcomes. The necessary changes identified by leaders creating a culture of transformation have included the following goals:

- Computerized documentation to minimize the need to interpret physician handwriting
- Streamlined documentation that can be completed by the nurse in less than 15 minutes for each shift
- Elimination of the need to ask a patient for the same information over and over
- Documentation of information only once, namely, allergies and past medical history
- An environment in which all employees provide nurturing, compassionate, respectful, creative, and excellent clinical patient care

- A patient care delivery model in which all caregivers are not only allowed but are expected to use their full scope of practice as defined by their licensure
- Equipment in the patient care area that supports patient lifting and minimizes nurse lifting
- Access to online reference sources, policies, and procedures, and a documentation system that alerts the caregiver to standards of patient care
- Adequate space for the family at the bedside
- The right computer device is available at the right time and in the right place for every patient
- Access to members of an interdisciplinary team on the patient care unit
- Ongoing research is conducted to validate processes and outcomes

It is important to note that none of these activities alone will transform the culture. Transformation will occur through the collective commitment to the majority of these behaviors.

Dare to Form New Partnerships

Leaders often wonder why we can't all just get along. Both external and internal divisions or separations of individuals, departments, organizations, and funding sources may make it difficult to work together to benefit the community at large. Facility competes with facility, for-profits compete with not-for-profits, and nurses compete with other nurses. In a recent, revolutionary move, two major competing universities in the same state agreed to collaborate for the benefit of the state's residents. After discussion by several courageous leaders, one very new to the state and willing to reverse and challenge existing assumptions, a new model for education was proposed that included a new medical campus to support the growing health needs of the community.

The new partnership reflects several behaviors that should indeed be emulated by others: reaching out beyond usual insular boundaries toward a world of expanded opportunities; discarding old baggage of "my way" and "your way" to "our way"; enhancement of the use of technology to support innovation and communication; and documentation of increased efficiencies and convenience to the citizens of the state. The reach for new levels of excellence emerges from many sources, both expected and unexpected, and always begins with the re-creation of relationships and reversal of some key assumptions.

Dare to be Politically Competent

Elected officials make decisions that directly affect the work of health-care leaders, often without knowledge of the pertinent issues and the impact of their decisions. In one state, for example, 3 of 90 legislators have previous health care experience; one is a registered nurse who has not practiced for 20 years, one is a licensed practical nurse working part-time in a physician's office, and the third a retired human resources executive. The hard reality is that most elected officials know little about health-care issues and need the sage advice of knowledgeable health-care professionals.

Energy and encouragement often are needed to develop relationships with elected officials in the district. Knowing those individuals who make decisions about allocations of revenues to health, the environment, transportation, and sanitation are certainly important, but decisions made

---

Discussion

New Partnerships for Nursing

Given the need to improve resource use, share expertise, and provide services to greater numbers of individuals, how can nursing contribute to the community?

Consider the following dyads in your group and identify ways that new and different relationships between the two could accomplish the above goals.

Schools of medicine and nursing

Community colleges and universities

Nurses and social workers

Retried nurses and working nurses

Professional sports teams and nursing homes

Banks and hospice facilities

specific to health-care regulations directly impact the work of nurses. The courageous leader asserts him- or herself to establish communication with elected officials and gives regular comments on issues of interest on a regular basis. The availability of webcasts of legislative sessions and the use of e-mail communication by the legislators provide opportunities for real-time monitoring and communication of pertinent issues. Involvement in the policy-making process may seem insignificant and one might think that one call or letter will not make a difference. However, when the policy maker is unfamiliar with the topic and you are the only one sending your comments, one voice can indeed make a significant difference.

Dare to Reverse Assumptions

Many practices and values related to hierarchal behaviors between levels of caregivers, the location of patient care services, and the role of the patient in the provision of services have changed significantly. The physician is no longer the captain of the ship, but rather is a member of the health-care team, with other disciplines owning their own practice as colleagues with the physician provider. Health-care services have moved from the location of the provider much closer to the location of the patient and more recently to remote locations connected via telemedicine clinics. The patient is no longer the recipient of the values and decisions of providers but is now expected to be the director of his or her care. Each of these changes has reversed the original assumptions of care, namely that only the physician could direct care, care is delivered at the location of the provider, and the team of providers controlled and directed the care received by the patient. The shifts in assumptions require health-care providers to learn new skills, deliver care in different locations, and communicate as facilitators of care rather than the director of care.

Another assumption that the courageous leader reverses is the notion that being in the middle between the organization and the patient is inescapable and problematic due to the conflicting values of the patient and the system. The courageous leader thrives in the role of the *in-between position*, between the patient and the health-care system; seeing it as the ideal position in which to be the translator and advocate for the patient in selecting and evaluating patient care services consistent with his or her own needs. The courageous nurse recognizes those situations in which the position between the system or other providers and the patient creates a moral dilemma and poses ethical challenges for the nurse and works to resolve the issues. Further, the nurse works to create better conditions in the future, to ensure that the different options are addressed prior to reaching the crisis point. The courageous nurse leader does not defer to the hierarchal position of the organization; the nurse assumes the role of communication facilitator and creator of the context for safe, patient-driven care.

Dare to Retire Retirement

Have you ever wondered what is significant about the age of 65? To be sure, it is optional to retire at 65 years of age and begin to claim Social Security benefits. As people live longer, as more work shifts to knowledge work and replaces physical work, and as the economy requires some to continue to work, new structures for work are needed. While it might be difficult to change the Social Security system quickly, there are some solutions worth considering so all those workers who wish to work beyond the age of 65 can do so without penalty or feelings of inadequacy. The courageous leader is challenged to adjust physically demanding jobs and create new roles that value the knowledge and experience of

---

Quantum Gem

Institutions falter when they invest too much in *what is* and too little in *what could be.*

Hamel & Valikangas, 2003

the older worker. The rationale is not only about addressing worker shortages; it is also about valuing the skills of individuals regardless of their age and allowing them to contribute when able.

According to Dychtwald, Erickson & Morison (2004), the long-standing human resource policies that favor youth and push out older workers is out of date and indeed is leaving a severe shortage of talented workers. To address the need for skills, knowledge, experience, and relationships, new models of employment that honor and recognize experience are needed. Efforts to decrease the bias against older workers, create new recruitment approaches that entice the older worker, and institute flexible scheduling are strategies surely to be welcomed by older workers as bona fide efforts to accommodate their changing physical capabilities.

Finally, courageous leaders must work with policy makers to modify the current retirement plans and allow for flexible retirement that pro-rates retirement benefits instead of the current all-or-nothing payment strategies. Much can be accomplished to assist the older generation in being more productive, useful and less bored—and this leads to better health and less use of health-care insurance benefits.

SUMMARY

Courageous Self-Care: Leader Time Out

Quantum leaders can neither dwell in the past nor revel in the present. The work of the leader requires courage to know the self as best as one is able to, to overcome the current obstacles to moving forward, and to take courageous action to cocreate the future that reflects emerging expectations, new knowledge, and new technology. The need for leader resilience, the phenomenon of capacity for continuous reconstruction rather than spells of success followed by failure, and so on require a strong emphasis on one's personal energy and ability to focus at the moment in time. No leader can be perfectly focused and energized to do the work that needs to be done every day. Leader *time out* is a practice that serves the effective leader well. It is always important to remember that making *no decisions* is often better than making partially-thought-out, emotionally-charged decisions.

Leader time out also allows the leader to reflect on his or her fit with the current organization, culture, and colleagues. It is a time to consider reinvesting in the work or deciding to change employment. The time to move on from one position to another is seldom planned or perfectly timed. When all efforts to reconcile the gap between the personal you and the outside organization are expended without sufficient success, the courageous leader recognizes what has been accomplished and begins another pathway in health-care leadership, not as a failure but as a lifelong learner of the work of health care. But what is most important is that the courageous leader must leave an organization when there is a disconnect between the leader's internal values and the values of the external world.

Courageous Leader Affirmation

I am able to take courageous, consistent, and appropriate management actions to overcome barriers to achieving my organization's mission.

Exercise 1 Changing Paradigms

Much evidence has been developed specific to the high cost of turnover, both financially and qualitatively. The employee-focused paradigm supports long-term employment as a vehicle to increased quality and lower costs through established relationships and organizational commitments. In the age of the knowledge worker, the value of retention is necessarily changed. Mobility of knowledge and competence is the norm rather than the exception. Workers thrive on mobility and thrive on learning new skills and team performance. Given this evolution, design a new employee management philosophy to support the new values and minimize or eliminate the previously valued paradigm.

In this chapter, seven behaviors to assist leaders in developing courage have been identified. These include:

- Rework the work
- Eliminate your job
- Live in the world of information technology
- Transform the culture
- Form new partnerships
- Be politically competent
- Reverse assumptions

Select two behaviors from the list, one in which you are most competent and one in which you are the least competent. With a colleague, address the following:

- Share the situations specific to the courageous behaviors.
- What behaviors made you feel competent?
- What behaviors/situations made you feel less than competent?
- Given the same situations, what can you do differently?

REFERENCES

Chinn, P. L. (2004). *Peace and power: Creative leadership for building community* (6th ed.). Sudbury, MA: Jones & Bartlett.

Dychtwald, K., Erickson, T., & Morison, B. (2004). It's time to retire retirement. *Harvard Business Review* 82(3), 48–57.

Emerick, L. (2004). *Nurse vigilance and practice breakdown: A study of relationships*. Unpublished master's thesis, University of Ohio, Columbus.

Frieberg, K., & Frieberg, J. (2004). How gutsy leaders blow the doors off business-as-usual. *Leader to Leader* 33, 32–37.

Hesselbein, F. (2004). Circles of inclusion. *Leader to Leader* 32, 4–6.

Houweling, L. (2004). Image, function and style: A history of the nursing uniform. *AJN* 104(4), 40–48.

Kennedy, H. (2000). A model of exemplary midwifery practice: results of a delphi study. *Journal of Midwifery and Women's Health* 45(1), 4–19.

Kuhn, T. (1996). *The structure of scientific revolutions* (3rd ed.). Chicago: University of Chicago.

Porter-O'Grady, T. (2003). Creators & dreamweavers: Building conspiracies for innovation. *Nurse Leader* 2(1), 30–32.

SUGGESTED READING

Blakeney, B. 2003. Nursing's Message to the world. *Creative Nursing*. Vol 9(3); 4–8.

Fairman, J. (1992). Watchful vigilance: Nursing care, technology, and the development of intensive care units. *Nursing Research* 41(1): 56–60.

Hamel, G., & Valikangas, L. (2003). The quest for resilience. *Harvard Business Review* 81(9), 52–63.

Hegyvery, S. T. (2004). New partnerships, new opportunities. *Journal of Nursing Scholarship* 1.Vol. 36(1).

Hramec, A. B. (2001). Reflections on being in the middle. *Nursing Outlook* 49, 254–257.

CHAPTER 10

Leadership and Care of the Self

CHAPTER OBJECTIVES:

Upon completion of this chapter, the reader will:

1. Define the issues affecting the personal role of the leader and the impact of those issues on the exercise of leadership.

2. Name at least three spiritual attributes that relate to the person of the leader and that affect the exercise of good leadership.

3. Identify specific and unique elements of the personal exercise of leadership that represent the leader's ability to manage the role through chaos, change, and challenging team dynamics.

INTRODUCTION

Leadership is demanding work. There is nothing in leadership that is inherently rewarding, nor does anything generate from leadership that guarantees a continuing level of commitment and energy in the role. In fact, there are many who suggest that leadership is more challenging than rewarding.

One of the first elements of self-focus for the leader relates to an understanding that the leader must be willing to play the key role in attending to the self's needs. Leaders cannot expect in their role any real defined support from followers, nor should they. When leaders look for nurturance and renewal from followers, they are often disappointed. It isn't that followers won't give positive feedback, support, or encouragement to the leader, but they are not required to do so. Leaders do not ask of those being led for support, agreement, or encouragement. While it is nice when that happens, expecting it is illegitimate.

As noted previously in this book, leaders simply have no friends. The expectation of leadership does not include under its rubric the notion of friendship. It is not that the person of the leader does not have friends; it is instead that the role does not demand friendship as a part of its exercise. Therefore the leader should not expect to get the encouragement, support, and validation that friendship can offer. The leader in this set of circumstances can feel very alone.

> ### Gem
>
> Leaders must reflect in their own roles the skills of self-care. Leaders cannot take care of others if they are unable to attend to their own needs. Modeling the ability to address one's own needs positively and with a high degree of balance is the best exemplar for the staff to do the same in their own professional lives.

Some Basic Rules for the Leader

- The buck stops here
- You're usually always alone
- Leaders have no friends
- Accountability begins here
- Others are watching you, not listening to you
- You either create or eliminate blame games
- It's about respect, not love
- You are partner, not parent

Remember

Wise leaders create coalitions and partnership with other leaders. The leader knows that the only kind of understandable leadership support one can get is from other leaders experiencing the same struggles in the exercise of leadership. Leaders do not seek support from their staff. It is not that support cannot be found there, but it is inappropriate to seek it there.

Ego Management

- Develop an accurate sense of self
- Find a good mentor or role model
- Check personal behavior with others
- Do a regular 360 evaluation
- Follow up personal conflicts quickly
- Create a personal development program
- Assess behavior against outcomes
- Separate the public from the private life
- Have interests other than work

In truth, leadership is a lonely exercise. The leader stands apart from all others because the role demands that this person be willing to confront, challenge, and engage others in ways that may not facilitate the development of personal relationships. Not only does the leader not have friends, the leader also often creates conditions that do not generate positive feelings toward the leader. This can make it very challenging for the leader and increases the leadership level of difficulty.

GETTING SUPPORT

While the expression of personal leadership may be a lonely experience, leaders do have support in the system. A leader is not alone in the role. Leaders share that role with others who are also experiencing the isolation, challenges, and lack of rewards in the expression of personal leadership.

It is the obligation of individual leaders to recognize the collective support that they have in the role from other leaders. Leaders must gather together to do more than simply undertake the business of the organization. The gathering of leaders should also include opportunities for support, growth and development, and encouragement in the role. It should be a time where leaders share their personal story of leadership, including what has and what has not worked. This can only occur in a collective framework in which the story of leadership is shared among the leadership community in a way that can be understood by those who share the same experience. Leaders must come to recognize that their strength lies with each other and that this horizontal leadership community provides the foundation for encouraging, supporting, and advancing the role of the leader.

What frequently occurs as people move into the role of leader is a higher level of competition emerging between and among individuals. Leadership is historically structured in its orientation and hierarchical in its expression. Often, those who ascend the leadership ladder bring with them characteristics that represent their own personal commitment to growth and development, advancing their careers, and affirming their personal impact on the organization.

Good leaders do not come without egos. The ego is a powerful human psychological tool that encourages us to develop a personal identity, a place in the world, a sense of self and person and expresses itself in individuality and in purpose. Balanced against other personality characteristics, the ego serves a sound purpose and helps the individual assertively address the vagaries and challenges of life in a complex world.

On the other hand, an out-of-control and poorly managed ego can create a great deal of difficulties in human expression and personal relationship. The undisciplined ego runs wild and creates conditions in which individuals sacrifice the values of relationship, integrity, human interaction, and friendship on the altar of personal advancement and gain. When that happens, individuals in this circumstance run through the organization as though everything was a personal fight, creating noise, continuous challenge, and, frequently, personal and relational pain. The challenge for leaders is to find balance between the personal need to grow and make a significant contribution and the ego's need to be individually recognized. Successful leaders must establish meaningful relationships to advance the interests of the organization and to build personal and professional relationships within the context of a positive workplace. This balance is often difficult to achieve. Yet it is one of the most powerful elements of the personal work of the leader and a part of the obligation the leader takes on in assuming the role.

In the 21st-century organization, much has been learned about how organizations work, the role of individuals, the characteristics of leadership, and the needs of both people and organized systems. Part of the challenge of that experience is the recognition that all individuals, regardless of what they do in a work system, have value, seek meaning, and want to fully participate in the life of the organization. Recognizing this, the leader should never operate in a way that diminishes or in any way slights the expression of these needs. All people in the workplace depend on a disciplined ego to be well-managed in terms of advancing the interests of the leader but also balanced against advancing the needs of those he or she leads and of the organization of which they are all members.

A primary challenge for the leader is the recognition of the varying degrees of ego management that must exist within the leadership role in an organization. Regardless of how the role is defined or how the organization uses it or defines it in its various leadership categories, there will be a wide variety of personal expressions of the role as it unfolds in the organization. Individual leaders should recognize this diversity as essentially healthy and should also be aware that there are times when the diversity of persons can serve as an opportunity to ameliorate the impact of the ego and keep it directed to a common purpose.

Part of the challenge is for leaders to comprehend in the 21st-century organization the differences between the categories of leadership that are not simply differentiated by level of leadership (organizational chart). This comprehension does two things: one, it helps the leader focus on the contribution of the role; and two, it helps the leader understand the value of the essential relationship between leaders in fulfilling the goals and objectives of the organization and the needs of those who provide its work. Every leader must recognize that every leadership role must make a contribution to the organization, regardless of where the position of leadership is expressed. The purpose of leadership, essentially, is to help the organizational community attain its mutually defined goals, achieve sustainability, and advance its interests with regard to its own future. Within the context of this understanding, every category of leader must contribute at some level to the values of the organization, to its purposes, and ultimately to achieving its goals. Therefore, whenever expressing the role of leadership, individual leaders should recognize that their specific role is always significant, valid, valuable, and important to the viability and sustainability of the organizational community.

This understanding of the role of leader should help the leader move away from a traditional view in a vertical orientation of leaders to other leaders. The old notion of leader as "boss" is one that is no longer viable and doesn't reflect the working of the human community network. The leader recognizes that he or she is playing a role that operates in the interests of the organization, to which that role has been directed. The leader understands that advancing the goals of the organization and assuring its success comes from the collective integration of the efforts of all leaders and those who do the work of the organization. It is this notion of collective intersection and interface that drives a clearer understanding of valuing and expressing the role of the leader.

Leaders must understand that they are differentiated from each other simply by their obligations to the organization. Each role has a fundamentally different impact driven by different requirements, depending on the role's position and application in the organization. Even with individual expectations, each role depends on the performance of other leadership roles in a way that assure the individual role is successful. No organization advances successfully upon a unilateral decision or action of the role of a single leader.

The Leader's Role

Leaders are defined by role, not by position. Regardless of where the role is located, it has specific contributions to make to the people and to the organization. The role is defined by that contribution, not by the position it represents. Everyone has a right to know what contribution the role makes to the organization. Defining positional status does not answer this question.

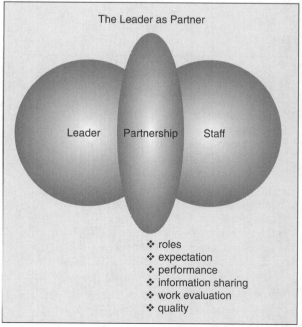

The Leader as Partner

Leader   Partnership   Staff

- ❖ roles
- ❖ expectation
- ❖ performance
- ❖ information sharing
- ❖ work evaluation
- ❖ quality

Critical understanding of the mutuality and intersection of leadership roles with regard to advancing the interests of the organization is critical to understanding organizational success. The individual leader must recognize her or his role within the context of collective leadership commitment, obligation, and purpose.

From this understanding, individual leaders come to recognize that a unilateral expression of ego at the expense of the relationship with the leadership team and others who do the work of the organization creates a deficit, not only for the organization and the achievement of its purposes but also for the exercise of individual and collective leadership. The ego-driven individual works at the expense of others and therefore fails to facilitate the relationships and interactions necessary for the collective action and wisdom of leadership.

The individual leader should bring to mind several things with regard to the balanced expression of good leadership. Each of these questions should be a part of the formation of the leader's intent in assuming the role and in expressing leadership on behalf of the organization. These questions essentially call the individual leader to discern purpose, reason, and intent for exercising the leadership role in a very personal way.

1. What personal need am I fulfilling by assuming the role of leader?
2. What satisfactions do I obtain from the expression of the role of leader?
3. What rewards am I receiving in the expression of this leadership role, and am I renewed by them?
4. How do I see my expression of this leadership role advancing the interests of the organization and the needs of those I lead?
5. How has the organization expressed what it needs from this role, and am I expressing the role as the organization sees it?
6. What difference do I think this leadership role will create for the organization?
7. What difference do I think this leadership role will make in my own life?
8. How will others' lives be better because of my exercise of this leadership role?
9. Have I written down my personal goals, needs, purposes, and expected accomplishments in my expression of this role of leader?
10. In what ways will I advance the role of other leaders in fulfilling the mission and purposes of the organization to which we are all mutually committed?

Remaining clear about one's own role and the need of that role in the expression of leadership provides a frame of reference that advances the meaning and value of the leadership role within the individual's life journey. Individuals who continually keep the above questions before them help to manage the vagaries of the ego, keep tabs on its action, and balance its force against the activities of service and purpose. Constantly attending to the need of creating an ego balance helps the individual leader keep the role in context, maintain the integrity of personal contribution, and ensure a continuing commitment to growth, development, and maturation as a good leader.

THE LEADER AS A LEARNER

Like any other pursuit, leadership is a journey. The only difference with regard to leadership is that leadership is a journey with no permanent destination. The journey that the leader represents is one of lasting commitment to personal growth, development, and improvement. What

---

Leadership and Mutuality

Leaders are in place in organizations to achieve organizational goals. The organization is not a vehicle for the leader to achieve unilateral goals. Leaders are recognized by the extent of their capacity to advance the interests of the organization and to create a high level of success. In addition, the leader extends the same enthusiasm and commitment to the minds and the work of the staff.

Leaders Are Always Testing Their Assumptions:

- about others
- about the organization
- about their role
- about individual effectiveness
- about expectations
- about understanding
- about individual responsibility
- about the direction of change
- about personal growth
- about achievement of goals

is critical for the leader is the recognition that the role requires continuous and endless personal growth and development.

No leadership role provides all that is necessary for the leader to succeed in it. The role can only be successful to the extent that there is goodness of fit between the skills of the leader and the demands of the role. This match, however, rarely occurs. Most leadership roles have demands that outstrip the ability of the leader living in the role. The vagaries and challenges of life in all of the experiences that it brings creates so much diversity and complexity that it often surpasses the skill level and the confidence of any leader, regardless of how much she or he knows and what that leader's role is in the organization.

The important issue is for the leader to acknowledge that he or she cannot know everything there is to know about the role. The more important concern is whether the leader is committed to learning and gaining insight from the expression of the role in circumstances and occasions when the demand is greater than the leader's individual skill. This is the real test of leadership.

It is not how much the leader knows. It is instead what the leader is willing to risk on the journey of development and growth in the expression of the role that is critical to effectiveness. As covered elsewhere in this book, issues of openness, vulnerability, risk taking, awareness, availability, and engagement in the role are all fundamental elements of the successful expression of the leadership role.

The leadership role reflects the journey of life. The leader is an exemplar of commitment to the full engagement of the life experience. The leader exemplifies a continuing and ongoing engagement of the vagaries and challenges of life and exemplifies in that role the willingness and ability to confront and address whatever issues life brings. They give witness for the expression of their role to those they lead, indicating thereby the appropriate mechanisms and responses to the challenges that confront all individuals in the expression of their life and their work. Leaders should exemplify the expression of the leadership role, acknowledging their openness to the unpredictability of the role and the many unfolding uncertainties and human and environmental challenges that create delight in its expression.

Leadership is not only found in the management of the rituals and routines of work. Simply engaging these routines and saying that they are successfully carried out does not signify effective leadership. In fact, managing these processes is not necessarily an expression of good leadership. This is not to suggest that good management is not necessary in undertaking the routine aspects of accomplishing work. It is. But it is important to understand that the leader's role goes beyond the basic expectations and that its expression is founded in how successfully the individual confronts those things that fall outside of the routine, challenge the normative, and raise expectations for performance. This is especially critical as the work environment continues to shift and change and increase in complexity. These many and varied situational shifts in the experience of life and work create a contextual framework for the expression of the role of leader. In fact these variables, these challenges, and the resulting noise in the organization are the meat of the work of the leader. It is these times and these circumstances that test leadership emergence and underpin the basic constructs for leadership performance.

CHAOS AND THE DEMAND FOR LEADERSHIP

Chaos provides an opportunity to understand the operation and workings of the universe as it applies to all human life. All the vagaries of

---

Leaders Never Stop Learning

Good leaders are continually growing. Development is fundamental to the role. The good leader is committed to personal growth and development, first in themselves and then in those they lead. The leader should not expect competence from the staff if the leader is not committed to personal continuing development.

Leadership Is a Journey

The good leader recognizes that leadership is a progressive and growth-driven experience. In short, it is a journey that never ends. The leader reflects this understanding within the role and acts as a beacon for those who are led so that they too might see the journey embedded in their own roles.

Innovation and Creativity

The work environment is continually shifting and changing, and the good leader is one who can accommodate that change. This leader:

- adapts quickly
- looks for subtle shifts
- reads the landscape well
- lives in the potential
- is always searching for more information
- has a diverse network of colleagues
- continuously communicates with others

chaos, the fundamental constituent of the universe, have an impact on every aspect of human existence. At the personal level, chaos affects the choices that we make, the way in which we live our lives, the opportunities that are available to us, and the outcomes that result from the variety of responses we give to any demand on our energy and resources. In short, "noise" is a synonym for the operation of chaos in our lives. Noise in this case means the incongruent and often unexplainable convergence of forces and factors that influence the thoughts and actions of an individual. While noise is consistent with the operation of chaos, it is not always comfortable in the context of individuals' lives. Noise represents the vagaries and inconsistencies of all processes of human experience. The wise leader, recognizing the operation of noise, functionally incorporates it into all interaction and communication.

These multidirectional and nonlinear energies associated with a quantum understanding of the universe become an important undercurrent in the expression of the role of the leader. The wise leader reflects on the reality and the permanence of noise and seeks to accommodate it through meaningful dialogue and effective processes. Early recognition that these quantum shifts and the related ebbs and flows often confound and confuse can guide the leader's thinking. The noise associated with this confusion creates a high level of incongruity and affects people's belief in their understanding and their rituals and routines. Most of the time, the leader will confront in others the pain and discomfort they feel in relationship to their own experience of chaos.

The leader must not only give evidence of accommodating the noise of chaos but also be able to exemplify a personal sense of calm in the acceptance and engagement of essential chaos. This is difficult if the leader has not concluded that confronting chaos is a fundamental constituent of the role, which is necessary for incorporating both an understanding of chaos and the ability to maximize the opportunities contained therein within the context of his or her own level of tolerance and acceptance.

Personal discomfort with uncertainty and the vagaries of change requires that the leader be able to reflect on his or her own personal accommodations to change. If the leader does not find adaptation to change consonant with personal expectations, it will be difficult to guide others into acceptance of their own change. This does not mean that the leader must be free from struggle or conflict associated with adjusting to major change. It does mean that the leader represents in personal behavior a willingness, openness, and engagement of the challenges, demands, and noise of change. It is this willingness that attests to and demonstrates the leader's personal engagement of the realities of change and a peaceful accommodation of their impact on the expression of the role.

This accommodation means that the leader undergoes reflection and personal dialogue, finding a place in the change experience where he or she can be at peace with the demands for change and the vagaries and inconsistencies of transformation in the chaos embedded in all change processes. Arriving at this point is not easy. What is critical for the leader is the ability to reflect personally on those forces and factors that affect her or his ability to accommodate the chaos and noise of quantum change. There are several factors that can influence the leader's accommodation and engagement of the personal challenges in addressing the experience of chaos:

1. *The willingness to look at life as a journey.* The wise leader engages the vagaries of change by recognizing the broader journey. This leader understands that life is a longer set of challenges that when looked at individually can overwhelm. However, when each chal-

lenge is looked at in the larger set of challenges and aggregated within the context of the life journey, each does not appear as daunting and overwhelming as it might without context. The leader begins to recognize that all processes in each element of the experience are dynamic, continuous, and endless. They are simply a portion of a longer journey that requires a deeper vision and more critical understanding of the link between individual action and the aggregated processes of life experience.

2. *The leader has developed highly refined reflective skills.* The ability to reflect, analyze, and evaluate individual occurrences within the context of larger occurrences is critical to the effectiveness of the expression of the leader's role and to helping others move through change. Leaders who react to change in the same fashion as their followers provide no real guidance or value to those followers. The followers have a right to expect that the leader has taken time to reflect on the issues confronting them, to have sorted through that which is viable and valuable and that which is not. Followers have a right to expect that the leader has taken all of the information and data with regard to change and has incorporated it into the larger journey in a way that is meaningful and valuable and contributes to mutual outcomes. The leader must be able to demonstrate that an accurate acknowledgment of the change process has been made, disciplined by a sound reflection of its context, its impact on the staff, and its ultimate impact on the goals and direction of the organization. This personal facility for reflection and for discernment is critical to the effectiveness of the leader's role in contemporary systems.

3. *The leader can translate the chaos of change into language followers understand.* As indicated in prior chapters, translation skills are important in the leader's toolbox. What is more important at the personal level is the leader's ability to translate the impact of change on his or her own life. As a team leader, there are always many challenges in implementing any change. What is important to the leader as an individual is an understanding of the demand of that change and a personal adaptation to incorporating that change within the context of the individual's own experience. Leaders should never ask followers to engage in change the leader has not already engaged. Leaders reflect in their behavior what they can expect to see in their own staff. At a personal level, the leader must be able to acknowledge the personal challenges, adaptations, and experiences of a given change so as to have already translated it into personal experience and applied it to accommodating behaviors. Through this process of lived leadership, the individual leader provides a framework out of which others can witness the leader's own struggle with change, and through positive experience, be able to adapt to the acceptance skills in the lives of each follower.

4. *Leaders love the future.* Leaders give followers an opportunity to hope. It is this commitment and belief in the possibility of the future that most exemplifies the positive experiences of life. This desire to be a part of creating the future, to be a designer, is the most powerful example of truly sustainable engagement. If the leader can represent these characteristics in his or her own role, they translate into acceptance in others.

5. *Leaders embrace all of the activities that relate to creating a desirable future.* Preferable futures rarely arrive on their own. People give their future form and substance. Leaders in highly changing circum-

---

Managing the Journey

The leader fits the particular experiences of unit, service, and department with the larger journey of the organization. This goodness of fit assures a seamless connection between person, team, and system. To do this the leader focuses on:

- translating goals into practices
- finding points of good fit between service and system
- engaging individuals toward organizational goals
- assuring internal service matches external culture
- individual performance fulfills organizational goals
- all team members are enthused in their work

Translating Chaos

Leaders make chaos understandable to all those they lead by:

- anticipating the changes
- discerning the impact
- participating in design
- telling the story
- sorting through the irrelevant
- defining meaning
- reducing "noise"
- gathering the stakeholders
- celebrating the moment

Lived Leadership

Leaders represent their own vulnerability to change and the challenges it brings. They continually exhibit to those they lead:

- constant readiness
- continuous presence to others
- willingness to explore
- embracing the challenge
- demonstrating uncertainty
- questioning everything
- creating good questions
- avoiding permanent answers
- exhibiting uncertainty
- engaging team members

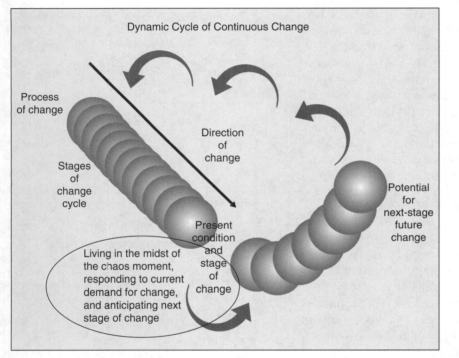

Dynamic Cycle of Continuous Change

Process of change

Direction of change

Stages of change cycle

Present condition and stage of change

Living in the midst of the chaos moment, responding to current demand for change, and anticipating next stage of change

Potential for next-stage future change

stances bear witness to the capacity to give personal form to the future so that followers may by example be able to do so in their own lives. The reflective and engaging leader stops momentarily to take stock of the impact of the change at the personal level and how that change has been translated into a way that can be reflected in the leader's behaviors. This reflected pattern of application becomes the behavior that staff see and for them exemplifies the appropriate lived application of the role to their own experience.

6. *Leaders overcome their individual fear of making bad choices.* The journey of change and moving toward the future always looks uncertain. Since the future has not been created simply because one sees it or discerns the direction toward it, its form and substance are still unclear. Whatever form the future will take depends on the individual response. There is always fear that the response will not match the demand. Leaders, however, exemplify a willingness to engage the risk of uncertainty and even failure in order to exemplify a willingness to embrace the construct, the elements that make up the journey to the future. This change process and the cycles of activities related to it calls the leader to make sense of the individual components and, subsequently, the integration of each component necessary to a successful change journey. This willingness to confront the challenges and face the vagaries of an unformed future model leads the staff to more appropriate patterns of response in their own behavior and makes it safe to confront their own issues. This modeling, this openness to uncertainties and risks, is more important in making meaningful change than even the skills and successes. Time, effort, gains, and losses will all impact the effectiveness of response and will either teach or direct leaders and followers about their failures or encourage them to be successful in unfolding essential change for themselves.

It is important for the leader to understand these processes as a part of the individual adaptation to change. It is the leader's behavior that has an impact on followers. If leaders cannot appropriately engage the demands of change through personal reflection, adaptation, and application, it cannot be expected that followers will be able to do so. It becomes critical for leaders to note at what level of doubt and personal courage they themselves are reacting to change and then model the level of safety for the staff in experiencing the same concerns. Whether the interpretation of the change is accurate or even appropriate, it is critical that the leader give evidence of comfort and confidence with regard to the vagaries of the quantum change process. Without this level of perceived comfort there can be no translation of ease in managing change to the staff. Without an internal sense of confidence, a good compass with regard to the direction of change, and a process for discernment and reflection, the leader cannot translate to the staff the behaviors or the insights appropriate to the accommodation of meaningful change.

PRINCIPLES OF UNCERTAINTY

The leader reflects in his or her own role the accommodation and acceptance of the characteristics and elements of uncertainty as a lived experience. The leader understands the following principles, which are always conditional within the exercise of leadership and have an impact on the behavior and expression of the role:

1. *The universe is a work in progress.* It continues to unfold and become. The universe is not a finished creation and, as such, represents the dynamic associated with "becoming." The leader, therefore, understands that individuals, organizations, systems, like the universe itself, are continually transforming and changing.

2. *Chaos and complexity are the essential constituents of the universe.* They do not go away; and they will never end. The universe can never be understood outside of its own condition of complexity, chaos, and uncertainty. This complexity and chaos as well as uncertainty relate to the endless "becoming" of the universe and the dynamic and inherent changes that unfold as a part of the complex interface of the array of factors acting in concert to influence whatever the universe will become.

3. *Everything in the universe is ultimately self-organizing.* All of the elements of the universe, including its patterns, mosaic, web, and intersections, create a framework requiring a high goodness of fit such that all of the elements work in concert to create the very next stage of change. This interconnectedness exemplifies the self-organizing and critical relationship existing at the intersection of all elements of the universe.

4. *Individuals, as a part of this universal constant, become co-creators of the future.* It is a willingness to deeply engage in the activities of transformation and change which empower individuals in the role of co-creation. Whatever generates from their effort is the form the future will take. This understanding that every individual influences the form and substance of change is important in valuing the process of change. At this level of understanding, change activities (or lack of them), when aggregated, create the conditions and circumstances that influence the form all change will ultimately take.

5. *All individuals, teams, organizations, and systems are smaller reflections of the totality of the universe.* In each individual, the complexity and dynamic of the entire universe are operating. The leader understands that the same dynamic of complexity, fluidity, and convergence is occurring at the local level as it unfolds in the entire universe. Therefore, every action, every person, every situation is, in one way or another, contributing to the aggregated action of the universe as it works to continuously and dynamically construct a future.

It is imperative for the leader to understand these principles as a fundamental constituent of the expression of the role of the leader. These principles and universal forces are acting continuously. It is through this ever-present movement of the universe with the confluence of human action that essential change is sustained. The success of the leader is directly determined by the competence of his or her own actions with the principles that guide the functions of change across the universal landscape.

The universe is unfinished work. So is the work of leadership. Leaders must never consider their work done. There is no measure of completeness; nothing is ever finished in the exercise of leadership. Leaders are "in play" the entire time that they are in the role. It is a role whose work is never done and whose task is never finished. Persons move through leadership, never complete it.

The Leader as Co-creator

The leader joins in the collective enterprise of creation, accessing and maximizing all resources, joining in the creative process, and working to create a sustainable future. Elements of co-creation:

- a comprehension of the integrity of all things
- empowering the collective wisdom
- recognizing the themes of change
- developing an aggregated vision
- translating vision into action
- encouraging and supporting others
- enumerating the meaning of everyone's contribution
- acknowledging and recognizing accomplishment
- keeping moving

Gem

It is important for the leader to understand the rules of complexity and the quantum processes operating in the universe. Just as these principles operate at the universal level, they also act at the individual level. The more the leader understands the action of complexity in all activities of human life and applies those principles to the process of leadership, the more effective the leader becomes.

LEADERSHIP AND CREATIVITY

It is vital for leaders to fully understand the expectations and functions of the role in light of knowledge generation and management. If the leader cannot live in the potential that is created in the tension between the present and future, it is likely the role will be compromised. Leaders must always demonstrate in their own role a personal pattern of positive response to the challenges of change invariably embedded in every aspect of leadership expression. Leaders must demonstrate in their own behavior that they have committed to fully engaging all of their resources in addressing change and the effort to create congruence between change and people's response to it. As the universe inevitably unfolds in undifferentiated and chaotic ways, yet represents a self-organizing facility, so must the leader demonstrate this same capacity. Since the universe evidences in every aspect of its unfolding the creative and innovative characteristics of uncertainty and of movement, so must the leader demonstrate her or his ability to positively embrace the challenges and vagaries of change. A level of joyfulness, even enthusiasm, must be exemplified within the context of the leader's role so that that enthusiasm can be contagious and evidenced in the roles of followers.

Enthusiasm

The leader must exemplify a level of energy and joy with regard to work and relationships. If the leader does not exemplify personal joy and happiness in the role of leader, there should be no expectation that joy and enthusiasm will be present in the role of the follower. Remember, leaders create context. The context created by the leader exemplifies the patterns of behavior that will be positively generated in the organization. A part of the challenge of creating good context is a personal joy and satisfaction leaders brings to their role and relationship with others. Somber and morose leaders can expect the same in their staff. If there is a clear engagement of the challenge and excitement of change present in the responses of the leader, it is likely that those behaviors will be present in the roles of the followers.

If the mental model for the role of the leader is that life is unfair, work is overbearing, and opportunities are nonexistent, it can be expected that will be reflected in the context that is created for the staff. The staff live the context that is provided for them in the role of the leader. The staff take their cue from the behavioral pattern of the leader and represent in their own behavior the mental model that the leader creates. It is therefore essential that the leader reflect in her or her his own role a level of joy and enthusiasm in confronting the opportunities and challenges of life. If the leader sees the journey of life as an opportunity for growth and advancement, it is likely staff will feel the same.

FOLLOWERS AS CO-CREATORS

Just as the leader represents a clear reflection of persons as co-creators in unfolding the future, the staff are co-creators with the leader in creating and providing substance for change. This notion of co-creator empowers followers to fully invest in the options and opportunities that derive out of their own role in creating a direction and response to the future. Co-creators are originators of the future, designers if you will, and in that role, begin to give the future whatever form it will take.

This is a powerful image. The leader creates this image in order to fully enable the followers to embrace the challenges of their own ex-

---

The Leadership Skill of Enthusiasm

- recognizing the positive forces of change
- telling the story of the larger journey of change
- a willingness to embrace the stages of life
- a personal aura of joy
- an infectious level of energy
- an ability to translate idea into action

Creating New Mental Models

Mental models reflect the way of thinking and of subsequently acting. They provide a context within which structure and behavior can unfold. The leader creates this frame for thinking and acting in order to encourage followers to give form and substance, resulting in an effective applied model. This work includes:

- the description of the change context for work
- articulation of the influences affecting work processes
- generating new rules affecting thinking and acting
- elucidating the impact of new concepts, technology, and applications
- stimulating others to identify creative response to changing circumstance

perience of change, both as individuals and as a team. This gives them full control over the circumstances and influences that result from their own choice and full participation. The leader communicates to the followers that full participation is an expectation of membership on the team and of their own personhood. Through that empowerment, the leader creates a level of intensity of response that ensures generativity, originality, and innovation in the team's movement toward creating their own future.

Chaos and the Need for Order

While chaos is an essential constituent of all change, it brings with it its own embedded sense of order. The order that we usually see in organizations really acts as a synonym for stability. While stability is desirable, it is also an inadequate notion. A certain level of personal stability needs to be present if the organization is to move confidently forward. However, stability should not be offered as a replacement for the challenges of transformation. Chaos brings with it a need for order. The kind of order that the leader provides is an order of confidence, support, presence, and continuity. The leader acts in the role of stabilizer by keeping the promise of presence, of faithfulness, of continuance with the workers in meeting the challenges of change. Stability comes from the constant confidence represented by the leader's encouragement, support, enthusiasm, information, and mobilization. This constant and consistent leadership support for the activities of the followers in the processes of creativity and innovation is the only stability and consistency necessary for effective change.

The Leader as Opportunity Creator

The leader as innovator and creator always sees the future through the eyes of opportunity. The leader becomes for the follower a living example of hope in the engagement of the future. Leadership becomes for those it influences a model of living in the potential, recognizing that the future is always open to the creative act. The person of the leader sees the future as a blank slate, an opportunity to give form and direction to human effort. The leader represents in her or his own behavior a full engagement of the range of resources and the creative processes necessary to ensure that the form change takes is meaningful and viable and makes a substantive difference to individuals and organizations.

Furthermore, leadership experience is not enough for the creative process. While experience is valuable, it does not in and of itself provide the full range of skills necessary to embrace and create a new future. Education and openness to learning is as necessary to effective and desirable future planning as is knowledge and experience. Experience is mostly about the past, reflective of those things already accomplished. It is insufficient as a tool for leaders to draw upon to give insights and information with regard to the direction of change. While experience can give the leader many sets of tools that he or she can use in anticipating changes, those tools are often not adequate in addressing the changes observed or the potential impact of those changes on individuals and organizations. Quite often new tools need to be created. Therefore, the leader embraces opportunities for new learning, new ways of thinking and seeing, creating and doing. Envisioning a new context tied to past experience helps the leader translate that vision into a plan of action and implementation.

Originality and Innovation

The leader values, indeed, treasures the creative impulse present in all people. The leader creates a context in which it is safe to experiment and to risk, allowing the staff to:

1. Attempt new approaches to old work
2. Identify new ways of working
3. Challenge existing policies and practices
4. Evaluate work processes for effectiveness
5. Bring in new reading, thinking, people to raise questions about existing practices

---

Creating New Opportunity

- identify ways of changing work
- allow the creation of new prototypes
- stimulate lateral thinking
- reward staff for innovation
- share credit with creators
- celebrate innovation often
- bring in new ideas, new reading
- set aside time for innovative conversation
- include other disciplines in creative dialogue
- create storyboards of new work processes
- present creative and innovative work to others

Putting Experience in Its Place

Experience is valuable. But it can also be a limitation. The wise leader is not held hostage to claims of experience. The leader knows that experience represents a validation of the past, of what has gone on before. In a time of critical and dramatic change, experience can become a serious impediment, crippling vision and taxing the creative impulse. We build on experience; we do not limit response because we have experience. Many organizations have died on the altar of experience as it precluded their availability to the transformative action of the new and innovative and impeded their ability to adapt.

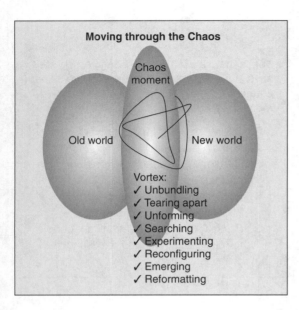

Moving through the Chaos

Chaos moment

Old world

New world

Vortex:
✓ Unbundling
✓ Tearing apart
✓ Unforming
✓ Searching
✓ Experimenting
✓ Reconfiguring
✓ Emerging
✓ Reformatting

Projecting a sense of self:

1. Clarity with regard to your own values
2. Understanding what the leader role means to you
3. Ability to put the role in the right context
4. Existence of a life outside of work
5. Evidence that you take time for yourself
6. Ability to hold firm to what you know is right
7. Willingness to advocate for what is true
8. Confidence in the exercise of one's role
9. Access to spiritual source of strength
10. Frequent self-renewal and time away

Living with Uncertainty and Mess

Change is messy. The leader, as indicated earlier, is comfortable with the mess and the noise of change and creates a place where others can be comfortable as well. However, just as important is the ability to confront the logical, systematic, organized, structured, and formal processes in the organization that themselves can act as an impediment to creativity and innovation. Also, the leader can personally impede creativity and change to the extent that he or she desires the stability and the safety of structure. In the old organization, formal structure is predicated against disarray and disorganization. Order was itself a desirable condition. In the midst of great change, order disappeared, as the ability to engender positive response out of the noise and messiness of change became critical to effective adaptation. In the midst of all change old structures and processes fall apart. Indeed, old structures are forced apart by those who are attempting to create an organized response to a demand for change in the organization. In the midst of such change, it is critical for the leader to be able to unbundle an attachment to order and to find embedded in the midst of a demand for change a creative response to the destructive process.

Positive destruction means purposely breaking apart or tearing down the organizational structures and systems in order to create the "vacuum" out of which new forms, structures, and systems can unfold. Without creating this opportunity for deconstruction, there is limited availability and openness for the new, the different, the innovative. The leader, understanding this dynamic, regularly examines current structures and organizational stability in an effort to challenge them when they impede new forms, structures, and innovations.

Leaders Always Preserves Their Sense of Self

In the midst of all of change and challenges of transformation, it is easy for the individual to lose a sense of identity and of personhood. The leader must always be aware of the struggle for identity in a changing organizational system. Understanding one's own role and meaning in undertaking change is critical to surviving it. Often individuals will identify that they have burned out because their work has changed. Work always changes. It can never remain constant. If one finds meaning in work, it is clear that one's meaning is located in the wrong place. Meaning drives work. Work is a reflection of value of purpose. If meaning becomes lost in the purpose of doing the work, the value of it gets lost, too.

It is often easy to embed one's identity within the context of work. When that happens and work changes, meaning and identity can become lost. The leader must periodically reflect in the course of his or her own activities on the meaning and purpose for those activities. As the activities themselves change, reflecting on the meaning of work and its purpose calls the leader to remain grounded in those values and principles that guide personal action and validate individual identity. Leaders who get swept up in the work of change and transformation frequently get lost in that work. As the work unfolds or as it gets completed, emotional dissatisfaction, depression, and even a lack of direction can sometimes emerge. The completion of work should not result in a loss of direction. Completing a particular job, task, or assignment does not mean that the work is ended. It means instead that the tasks associated with the continuum of transformation in change have moved on to demand a different response and unique set of emergent activities. Remaining in touch with one's meaning allows the vagaries and inconsistencies associated with changing and transforming work to continue to stimulate change without threatening value and meaning over the course of that change. Keeping in touch with this purpose and meaning ensures for the leader a grounding in values and the representation of the sustainability of personal principal. Good leaders always act in concert with the team.

Individual Action Cannot Stand Alone

In moving toward meaningful change, the collective energies and efforts of all are necessary to create sustainability in the change. The leader guides all members of the team in a common direction committed to achieving aggregated value for the team and for the purposes the team is directed to fulfill. All change operates within the context of team values. The leader recognizes that if the organization changes, its people have also changed. The rules, processes, conditions, and elements of growing and changing act both individually and collectively. Whatever its work, the team moves ahead, acting in concert and working together to create the conditions of living in a new way and acting in a new place.

The Leader Constantly Assesses His or Her Relationship With the Team

The intensity of the leader's relationship and the quality of the interaction is a determinant of the success of the work of the organization. Since most of that work is accomplished through effective team action, the leader is critically aware that his or her efforts guide the organization to sustainable success. Discernment is a greater gift than definition. The leader constantly reflects on the relational needs of the team, the needs of individuals, even the need of the leader in relationship to his or her team. Leaders must recognize that they need from their team a sense of support, affiliation, and renewal, just as the team needs that from the leader. The leader must make this known to the team. This is a collaborative relationship. The ebbs and flows of personal interaction and collective action have as much impact on the leader as it does on the team. The person of the leader needs an opportunity for expression, communication affiliation, and collective action with a full understanding that those integrated activities can lead to both individual and group success. Therefore, the leader must make clear to team members the leader's needs in terms of communication, interaction, support, and performance from followers. Fulfilling the individual leader's needs as well as attending to the followers' needs creates a dynamic of interaction and intersection between leader and team that is essential to maintaining the energy and the commitment to continuous and dynamic change.

Leadership Work is Not Easy Work

No one should stay in the role of leader without a clear and discerning understanding of the implications of the exercise of leadership. All of the demands of leadership and the needs of the leader must be carefully considered every moment that leadership is being expressed. The person of the leader is like any other individual in the organization. This person has strengths and weaknesses, good moments and bad moments, ups and downs, all of which influence the effectiveness of the leader's expression of the role. The leader must attend to the person inside and address whatever specific individual needs give reason, value, and meaning for exercising the role. Continuous and constant reflection of the role, the dynamics influencing the expression of the role, the relationships

---

Sustaining a Sense of Direction

The leader recognizes that any particular work falls within the context of a greater concert. Occasionally "going to the balcony" provides the leader an opportunity to develop a broader and deeper insight with regard to the context of change affecting the activities and practices of daily work. The leader regularly visits the balcony to see work at a longer distance, translate the journey in broader terms, instill meaning in the activities of the worker, and deepen the sense of meaning for all members of the team.

Effective Leaders Always Work through Teams

Leaders are continually working with groups, attempting to move many people through the process of change and innovation. Therefore, team skills are an important fundamental for all leadership roles. Leaders need to understand:

- Work always gets done through teams
- Teams require a lot of horizontal communication
- Teams need good information
- Teams are always looking for encouragement
- All teams experience conflict
- Facilitating teams requires great group skills
- Leaders must constantly remind teams of goals
- The major leader's work is maintaining team relationships
- Team outcomes are more sustainable than individual results

Team Culture

All teams have their unique characteristics. The wise leader assesses the particular communication, relationship, and interactional dynamics of individual teams, and through that process, begins to understand the team's personal identity. That identity is unique to the team and informs the leader what will work best in motivating and leading that team.

Leadership Is Never Easy Work

The leader recognizes that the demands of leadership are ever-changing, depending on the circumstances and the need of the team and the goals of the organization.

Organizations are dynamic entities, constantly in motion, requiring continuous reevaluation and reconfiguration of the efforts of work around ever-changing goals. This creates emotional demand on both leader and follower, increasing the need for support, time away from work, rest, and relaxation.

Gem

Leaders simply cannot maintain the energy necessary to the role without a mechanism of renewal and regeneration. Whatever the spiritual values that lie at the heart of the individual leader's personal principles, they need to act as a source of reflection and regeneration. A leader with no spiritual center is a leader who acts with no soul.

Gem

Leaders are always advocates. That can sometimes position the leader to act individually, swim upstream, confront organizational leadership, create team discomfort, and slow progress. The courageous leader recognizes these times will occasionally arise and will call for personal commitment, energy, and clarity in helping the organization perceive that which is most difficult yet essential to its own growth.

necessary to maintaining the energy and commitment in the role, and the personal challenges and facilities the individual brings to the role must be renewed if there is to be any success in the expression of leadership.

SPIRITUAL INTELLIGENCE: FINDING THE COURAGE WITHIN

Spiritual integrity is an essential component of good leadership expression. Leadership is not simply a set of skills but is in fact a discipline. The term "discipline" means that leadership has its own set of rules and characteristics, demands, and criteria for its appropriate and sustainable expression. Leaders must express the role, not only to lead and direct the process of change but also to create the conditions by which change itself is experienced by others. Therefore, the leader is intimately aware of the impact of change on the leader's own person and confronts that impact with openness and personal availability. The leader must be able to adapt to the change and exemplify adaptability and fluidity in meeting the demands and the vagaries of shifting work obligations. Leaders, therefore, are always involved in seeking and reaching their own potential.

Leaders cannot, however, reach their potential without reflecting deeply on their own relationship to life and to their own personal spiritual journey. Leadership demands great courage and persistence. It confronts high elements of risk and of pervasive challenge. Leaders are constantly living in a potential between current reality and the unfolding future. This is a place of great demand and risk. The leader is called to translate the potential into a language that followers can understand. In order to do this, the leader must be able to understand the potential within his or her own experience and give it a personal language so that it has meaning in the self-expression of the role. Leaders are always making others aware of meaning and purpose in change and help others ultimately seek the direction necessary to achieve meaningful change. As a result, leaders must live on the cutting edge; they must constantly be "pushing the boundaries" of consciousness and of innovation. Leaders focus the staff's energies on confronting their own behaviors, perceptions, and actions in relationship to the change process. In order to do this successfully, leaders must be clear through their own expression of leadership about what the change means, the direction of that change, and the value of that change as a part of their own personal leadership expression.

Leaders are often on the cutting edge of change. When one is on the cutting edge of change, there is limited support, sometimes even limited understanding, with regard to the change. The leader is often looked at as an anomaly, perhaps as an organizational "pain," and as a result doesn't have much support even perhaps from followers. Having confronted the vagaries and challenges of change and the independence needed to undertake meaningful change, the leader comes to more clearly accept the fact that leadership is often a lonely experience. However, being in touch with the spiritual values in the expression of that role and recognizing the essential loneliness of the role can cause the leader to draw on spiritual resources, which can be a source of strength.

The leader recognizes that he or she cannot take care of others if they cannot take care of themselves. Self-sacrifice, abandonment of individuality, or being long-suffering or passive are mindless energies that can take over if the leader is not fully aware of the values and purposes for undertaking any particular action. Good leaders have a strong sense of their own identity and values and stay completely in touch with those motives and intentions that relate or exemplify the values that lie at the core of their own leadership. Leaders recognize the essential elements and characteristics of change, are able to identify where individuals and organizations are in their transition to change, and are able to identify the most appropriate responses in any given time and place. Here again, time for reflection, discernment, exploration, and clarification are all elements of the leader's spiritual skill set. The leader will draw on the conclusions and assessments made in moments of reflection and will make choices that reflect deeper meaning and ultimately respect the connection with the self that indicates the leader's ability to understand, willingness to risk, and expression of energy necessary to engage and undertake successful change.

Fundamental Leadership Elements

Spiritual integrity

Personal competence

Effective relationships

Shifting Contextual Circumstances

> constantly moving universe
> shifting world of work
> consistently constrained resources
> challenging people's personalities
> worker behavior inconsistencies
> fast pace of change
> changing demand of market and "users"
> constantly new and transforming information

The universe is full of mystery and creative uncertainty. The leader's individual personal beliefs and traditions bring the leader to understand that the universe is full of mystery, uncertainty, and many challenges to change. Most of our beliefs accommodate those things we do not know. However as we become clearer about what we can know, that knowledge can confront the very beliefs that are central to our fundamental value system. Here again, the leader is open to challenge and to exploring what knowledge does in terms of beliefs and past practices. Knowledge should reflect light into our beliefs so that we do not hold blindly onto those that knowledge can easily address, challenge, and change.

The leader should always remember that the universe is in continuous motion, constantly shifting and adapting and changing its own form and direction. Still, deeply embedded is a sense of order and "systemness" that reflects a set of principles and processes that are as ancient as creation and as contemporary as the latest creative act. No change happens simply for its own sake. All change is a reflection of the greater concert, such that when linked with all other efforts it creates a symphony or mosaic that ultimately deepens the picture of understanding that we have of the change itself. Our beliefs should not be so rigid and so fixed that the revelation of science and the generation of new knowledge cannot inform and advance our beliefs. This is as much a part of the spiritual journey as any other element.

What is also important is to respect the value of prayer, whatever that might reflect for the leader. There are many kinds of religious and spiritual practices that an individual can draw on in terms of expressing meaning and value through prayer. Whatever that tradition is for the leader, it should encourage and strengthened the individual, help realign the individual's energies and principles, and continuously motivate the individual to seek higher levels of performance and to advance individual and collective levels of understanding and application. However prayer renews, strengthens, and encourages, it should refresh the individual and renew individual effort in the leadership role and in meeting the challenges of change.

Finally, the leader exemplifies in the context of his or her own role a clear understanding that all efforts, regardless of whether they are related to work or home, are all part of a larger journey of transformation change and growth. The leader reflects the challenges of expressing the role of the leader, substantiating that all change is normal and should be expected as a fundamental part of the exercise of work. Translating this within the context of one's own efforts creates for the leader the primary drive for the role in relationship to those she or he leads. People can change by design or by default. It is a requisite of the leader to help during change by designing so that others are not affected in a negative way,

---

Leadership and Mystery

Not everything can be knowable or understandable at once. The leader recognizes that, embedded in every activity, change and possibility are elements of uncertainty that reflect the unknowing and mystery embedded in all human experience. The leader comes to appreciate the value of this finding and sees it as a representation of the eternal curiosity that continues to motivate, encourage and inspire.

Gem

The transforming leader comes to understand the leader's work as a part of a great opus. The leader recognizes in everyone's effort an individual contribution to a greater effort that when aggregated to all efforts contributes to the dance of the universe, advancing, revealing, renewing, and enhancing all of human experience. No matter how small the effort, it is an essential contributor to the mosaic of the living universe.

having failed to see the implications and actions of change soon enough for it to make a difference in their own lives. Therefore the discernment of potential change is a critical element in the role of the leader. By applying the skill of understanding and translation, the leader is able to give a voice to change, its meaning, and its application in the lives of all those he or she meets. To do this, the leader must be in touch with this dynamic within her or his own person.

The leader is a creator. As a creator she or he joins the other creators, regardless of their location in the organization, to build a frame for the creative journey in the movement toward innovation and adaptation in organizations and in people. No one can provide the meaning and value for other individuals with strength and courage if the meaning and value is unable to emerge within the context of that individual's life. Imagine the number of leaders working in the world who use the role as the exercise of their own inadequacies. How many leaders attempt to obtain the role for power, ego renewal, personal support, and adulation? Leaders who need the role for these purposes end up using it as a personal vehicle rather than an opportunity for organizational and team creativity and advancement. Often these people need the role more than the role needs them.

The journey of leadership, like the journey of life, should be an experience that is without boundaries. Leadership is life lived in the white spaces, between the lines. In this place, the leader recognizes that the work is to create an opportunity, a frame of reference, a contextual framework where others are free to create, relate, grow, and advance, both as persons and as the organization. The leader accurately reads the signposts of the journey, translates them in a language that others can understand, and then joins with those willing to engage the journey in a meaningful experience that helps create the future. To do this, the leader must be able to engage personally, have a spiritual depth and a sense of purpose and continuous renewal. The leader must set aside time for the self, the spirit, and the energy renewal necessary to continue the process of leadership. This spiritual and personal transformation is a continuous dynamic that calls the leader to an ever-unfolding dance between present and future, personal and collective, and real and potential.

In the final analysis, the leader cannot create change in others if she or he cannot engage that same change within. This ability to identify with both change and followers is an important criteria for the measurement of great leadership. Leaders must attend to their own needs, but only in the context of how those needs ultimately serve the greater good of those they lead. Self-care, self-assessment, translation of leadership skills into the language of others, and joining of all human energy in the creative act of building a preferable future is the best testament to success in the role.

The Creative Leader

Leaders are the purveyors, stimulators, energizers of organized creativity. Therefore, the leader must exemplify the creative spirit:

- a love of play
- a little craziness
- affection for experimentation
- enjoys game-playing
- translates idea into action
- encourages different thinking
- creates a safe space
- allows others to innovate
- sees life as opportunity

Time Is Not the Enemy

Good leaders recognize that time is a gift, not a weapon. One major gift of human life is the ability for people to control their use of time. Time is a gift, a tool, a talent, nothing more. Leaders recognize that how time is used is a universal issue and the proper use of time is the greatest vehicle for creativity, innovation, and the full experience of life.

SUGGESTED READINGS

1. Allcorn, S. (2002). *Death of the spirit in the American workplace*. Westport, CT: Quorum Books. xxvii, 189.
2. Bar-On, R., & Parker, J. D. A.(2000). *The handbook of emotional intelligence: theory, development, assessment, and application at home, school, and in the workplace*. 1st ed. San Francisco, CA: Jossey-Bass. xv, 528.
3. Conger, J. A. (1994). *Spirit at work: discovering the spirituality in leadership*. 1st ed. San Francisco, CA: Jossey-Bass. xxxi, 222.
4. Giacalone, R. A., & Jurkiewicz, C. L. (2003). *Handbook of workplace spirituality and organizational performance*. Armonk, NY: M.E. Sharpe. xvi, 524.
5. Kalakota, R. & Robinson, M. (2001). *E-business 2.0: roadmap for success*. Addison-Wesley information technology series. Boston, MA: Addison-Wesley. xxiv, 520.
6. Kennedy, S. (1975). *Nurturing corporate images: total communication or ego trip?* Cranfield, England: Cranfield Institute Press for the School of Management. 39–83.
7. Kilmann, R. H., & Kilmann, I. (1994). *Managing ego energy: the transformation of personal meaning into organizational success*. 1st ed. Jossey-Bass management series. San Francisco, CA: Jossey-Bass. xxviii, 342.

8. Kincaid, J. W. (2003). *Customer relationship management*. Getting it right. Upper Saddle River, NJ: Prentice Hall PTR. xxvii, 480.

9. Mitroff, I. I. (2004). *Crisis leadership: planning for the unthinkable*. Hoboken, NJ: Wiley. xv, 121.

10. Owen, H. (1999). *The spirit of leadership: liberating the leader in each of us*. 1st ed. San Francisco, CA: Berrett-Koehler. vii, 156.

11. Rubin, H. (2002). *Collaborative leadership: developing effective partnerships in communities and schools*. Thousand Oaks, CA: Corwin Press. xviii, 111.

12. Spitzer, R. J. (2000). *The spirit of leadership: optimizing creativity and change in organizations*. Provo, UT: Executive Excellence Pub. 344.

SCENARIO 1: COMFORT WITH CHAOS

Jane sat in the strategy meeting and began to feel the rising pressure of tension within. The hospital was outlining a whole new direction for clinical services. This meeting involved establishing a different framework for the delivery of clinical services and was reemphasizing mobility-based and outpatient clinical services in place of the past focus of inpatient clinical care. For Jane, this meant a complete shift in the service structure and orientation of her clinical unit. Her concern was heightened as she reflected on a recent shift in the focus of her clinical service and the reorientation of the medical staff to different models of medical care. On top of this change, a new electronic medical record had been introduced and the clinical staff was struggling with adapting to documenting and recording of care in that new model. New challenges with regard to quality priorities had also been initiated in the past year, calling all clinical providers to refocus their activities using a new quality format that would better document clinical process and the achievement of outcomes. In addition, a new staffing and workload management system was being introduced in order to better undertake patient care assignments, distribute staff across the shifts, and initiate better control mechanisms with regard to the use of overtime. Jane was beginning to have feelings of panic, a sense of being overwhelmed by the pace and the complexity of change. She didn't know if she could continue to cope. If she couldn't continue to cope, Jane wondered, how in the world will the staff be able to handle this level of intensity of change: And how would Jane lead them through it?

Scenario exploration:

As a learning team discuss together in detail the following questions:

1. Is this the pace of change in today's health-care environment?
2. Are leaders today becoming overwhelmed with the rate and pace of change?
3. Are the number of changes that are occurring in today's world too much for leaders and workers to handle in the workplace?

Following the exploration of these questions, break up into small groups and explore the following questions in relationship to Jane's experience of change:

1. What has caused Jane to feel particularly overwhelmed as a leader?
2. What is Jane's best first response to the feelings she is currently experiencing?
3. Is Jane capable of dealing with the level of complexity that leadership now requires, or should she change roles?
4. How we do break down and establish priorities for how Jane might approach her issues of complexity?
5. What advice would you give Jane in dealing with workplace issues and leading staff through the complexity of change?

continues

SCENARIO- 1: COMFORT WITH CHAOS *continued*

Following the small group process and response to the above questions, regather in a larger group and share by comparing and contrasting your responses. At the completion of your dialogue, construct a leadership charter that would guide the leader in establishing a set of principles and priorities in living in a time of complexity and chaos and leading others through it. Reflect on the group charter, and as individuals, construct a personal leadership charter that will guide your own leadership development and application as you unfold your own leadership role.

SCENARIO 2: BECOMING OVERWHELMED

Nora has been the department manager for some 10 years. She is a good manager. Lots had been accomplished over the past 10 years as the technology of the service advanced and as clinical practice improved. Patient care had advanced, length of stay had declined, therapeutic intervention had been highly successful, and patient satisfaction scores had remained consistently high. Much had been accomplished.

Yet, Nora felt depressed with a decreasing level of energy. She had worked hard over the past 10 years, taking little time for herself in order to build the department to the level of success it had achieved. She found the work exciting and energizing and found every opportunity to be creative and innovative in building this new service. Her work was her source of energy and satisfaction. Nora felt she did not need to take weeks of vacation like so many other people. She saw her work as fun, constantly energizing her, acting as a source of creativity and of joy. Lately, however, joy had been missing. Her energy didn't seem to operate at as a high a level. She still found the work satisfying and energizing, but something seemed to be missing. The pace of change seem to overwhelm more than it used to. Staff complaints seem to irritate her more than they did in the past. She couldn't quite understand what was happening with her and what quite to do about it.

Scenario exploration:

In reviewing the scenario, break up into teams of four to five members. In your team, process and respond to the following questions:

1. What are your feelings about Nora's work practices?
2. Was Nora's satisfaction with the challenges of her work sufficient to encourage, renew, and motivate her?
3. How did Nora renew herself, and was it sufficient to sustain her?
4. What three things in your judgment did Nora ignore or fail to recognize in her approach to leadership?
5. At this stage in Nora's circumstances, what would you recommend that she do?

After completion of your individual team sessions, rejoin with a larger group and compare your responses to the above questions. After completion of the discussion together, break into smaller groups again and undertake a role play with one member playing Nora's role and another acting as mentor to Nora, guiding and advising her with regard to what she might do with her circumstances. Pay special emphasis on helping Nora to develop personal insights and skills in relationship to her own leadership self-care and support.

Index